MOTIVATIONAL INTERVIEWING IN LIFE AND HEALTH COACHING

Applications of Motivational Interviewing

Stephen Rollnick, William R. Miller, and Theresa B. Moyers, Series Editors

Since the publication of Miller and Rollnick's classic *Motivational Interviewing*, now in its fourth edition, MI has been widely adopted as a tool for facilitating change. This highly practical series includes general MI resources as well as books on specific clinical contexts, problems, and populations. Each volume presents powerful MI strategies that are grounded in research and illustrated with concrete, "how-to-do-it" examples.

RECENT VOLUMES

Motivational Interviewing with Offenders:
Engagement, Rehabilitation, and Reentry
Jill D. Stinson and Michael D. Clark

Motivational Interviewing and CBT:
Combining Strategies for Maximum Effectiveness
Sylvie Naar and Steven A. Safren

Building Motivational Interviewing Skills:
A Practitioner Workbook, Second Edition
David B. Rosengren

Coaching Athletes to Be Their Best:
Motivational Interviewing in Sports
Stephen Rollnick, Jonathan Fader, Jeff Breckon, and Theresa B. Moyers

Motivational Interviewing for Leaders in the Helping Professions:
Facilitating Change in Organizations
Colleen Marshall and Anette Søgaard Nielsen

Motivational Interviewing in Social Work Practice, Second Edition
Melinda Hohman

Motivational Interviewing with Adolescents and Young Adults, Second Edition
Sylvie Naar and Mariann Suarez

Motivational Interviewing in Health Care, Second Edition:
Helping Patients Change Behavior
Stephen Rollnick, William R. Miller, and Christopher C. Butler

Motivational Interviewing, Fourth Edition:
Helping People Change and Grow
William R. Miller and Stephen Rollnick

Motivational Interviewing in Life and Health Coaching:
A Guide to Effective Practice
Cecilia H. Lanier, Patty Bean, and Stacey C. Arnold

MOTIVATIONAL INTERVIEWING in Life and Health Coaching

A Guide to Effective Practice

Cecilia H. Lanier
Patty Bean
Stacey C. Arnold

Series Editor's Note by William R. Miller

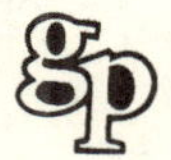

THE GUILFORD PRESS
New York London

A Division of Guilford Publications, Inc.
www.guilford.com

Printed in the United States of America

This book is printed on acid-free paper.

The authors have checked with sources believed to be reliable in their efforts to provide information that is complete and generally in accord with the standards of practice that are accepted at the time of publication. However, in view of the possibility of human error or changes in behavioral, mental health, or medical sciences, neither the authors, nor the editors and publisher, nor any other party who has been involved in the preparation or publication of this work warrants that the information contained herein is in every respect accurate or complete, and they are not responsible for any errors or omissions or the results obtained from the use of such information. Readers are encouraged to confirm the information contained in this book with other sources.

For product and safety concerns within the EU, please contact *GPSR@taylorandfrancis.com*, Taylor & Francis Verlag GmbH, Kaufingerstraße 24, 80331 München, Germany.

Last digit is print number: 9 8 7 6 5 4

Library of Congress Cataloging-in-Publication Data is available from the publisher.

ISBN 978-1-4625-5514-7 (paperback)
ISBN 978-1-4625-5515-4 (cloth)

To my husband, Bill, my patient listener for 46 years,
who has heard countless hours of my ideas
shared over our kitchen island;
and to my children, David and Lydia,
their spouses, Anna and Denney,
and my seven grandchildren,
who inspire me and remind me
not to take myself too seriously.
You all are my motivation.

—Cecilia H. Lanier

To the memory of my son, Adam;
to my husband, Dave, for his unwavering love and support;
and to my family members Joyce, Logan, Audrey,
Nicky, Jaelynn, Bailey, Payton, Maggie, Margaret, and Doug.
I am deeply grateful for your presence in my life and for the love,
laughter, adventure, positivity, and resilience that we share.

—Patty Bean

To my loving husband,
you are my confidant and greatest supporter;
and to my parents' enduring love
and the values you instilled in me.

—Stacey C. Arnold

About the Authors

Cecilia Lanier, MEd, is a National Board-Certified Health and Wellness Coach, a Functional Medicine Certified Health Coach in private practice in Alabama, and a course facilitator at the Functional Medicine Coaching Academy. With 25 years of experience as an educator, Ms. Lanier found her deepest passion in coaching fellow teachers during the final years of her teaching career. Motivational interviewing is the primary influence in her work.

Patty Bean is a Nebraska-based, Internal Family Systems-informed coach and licensed massage therapist in private practice. She is certified as a Master Wayfinder Life Coach, a Professional Certified Coach of the International Coaching Federation, a National Board-Certified Health and Wellness Coach, and a Functional Medicine Certified Health Coach. She has worked as a course facilitator at the Functional Medicine Coaching Academy. In addition to her coaching work, Ms. Bean teaches online QiGong, meditation, and yoga classes.

Stacey C. Arnold is a Functional Medicine Certified Health Coach and National Board-Certified Health and Wellness Coach in private practice in Georgia. She is also a certified personal trainer and certified Dietary Supplement Specialist, and an experienced organic gardener. In her coaching practice, Ms. Arnold has particular interests in gut health and sustainable, healthy living. Before becoming a coach, her professional experience included working in real estate and human resources.

Series Editor's Note

When Steve Rollnick and I wrote the original edition of *Motivational Interviewing* (MI) in 1991, we thought of it just as a tool for counselors and psychotherapists to use in treating people with substance use problems. A decade later, however, when it was time for our second edition to be published, it was already clear that MI was being applied in a broader array of helping professions by people who did not think of themselves as psychotherapists. MI was no longer just about addictions and was being used in medical and nursing care, nutritional counseling, probation, public health interventions, with parents, and on college campuses and in emergency rooms. For two more decades that trend has continued with applications of MI in leadership and management, sports coaching, education, veterinary care, social work, preventive dentistry, and farming. The person-centered approach of MI seems to be useful in many areas of human interaction.

Then in 2021, Theresa Moyers and I reviewed 70 years of psychological research to answer a vexing question: Why is it some counselors are so much more effective than others, even when delivering what seems to be the same treatment? We came up with eight characteristics of more effective therapists, whose clients are more likely to show positive change. After we published *Effective Psychotherapists,* it struck me that seven of these eight characteristics of more effective counselors have been part of MI from the very beginning, and the eighth should have been. Is that perhaps what we have been studying and teaching for 40 years—what makes helpers more helpful?

Though MI was initially developed within the realm of psychotherapy, it seems to be a way of having helpful conversations about change in a broad range of helping professions. It is firmly grounded in the person-centered approach of Carl Rogers, which itself has been applied broadly beyond psychotherapy in peacemaking, pastoral care, and education. It was a short step, then, to consider how MI can be an approach in the coaching professions, and here is the first text on this subject. Its authors explain how "the coach approach" closely resembles MI and vice versa. This is a "how-to" of the coach approach, consistent with the profession's professional and ethical standards.

There is a large scientific literature on MI in general, with over 2,000 controlled trials published, although studies of the efficacy of MI specifically in coaching are still in a relatively early stage and there is much to learn. The authors have focused on the possibilities of MI in the coaching professions while being careful not to step beyond the current science. I see important potential with MI to more carefully specify what coaches do and how it helps their clients make the positive changes they seek. A melding with MI may more generally help the coaching professions to develop quality assurance and outcome research.

I am personally pleased, then, with The Guilford Press publication of this first text on MI in coaching. It will be fascinating to see the fruits of this book. When our own first edition of *Motivational Interviewing* was published by Guilford over 30 years ago, we had little idea of what lay ahead. May you, readers, find here some tools and insights to enrich your own coaching and increase its benefits for those you seek to guide.

WILLIAM R. MILLER, PhD
University of New Mexico

Preface

Motivational interviewing (MI) has been adopted across numerous personal and professional settings, and now its influence has spread to the broader field of life coaching and various subspecialties, such as health and wellness coaching. During our training in life and health and wellness coaching, we noticed more than a few similarities between MI and professional coaching and wondered if MI was indeed a foundation for coaching. Did others see the clear parallels between the two professions, and if so, would learning and teaching MI help us and coach trainees become more effective coaches? We devoted ourselves to confirming this proposition, and this book is the result. We are not the first to notice how MI weaves perfectly into the professional coaching paradigm. The National Board for Health and Wellness Coaching echoes the MI approach, methods, and skills in its competencies and practical skills guidelines, which are used in coach-training programs. The tenets of MI also parallel the International Coaching Federation competencies for life coaching, considered the gold standard for professional coaching practice.

A deep-dive comparison of this type of professional coaching and MI confirmed our suspicion that coaching has its roots in MI. Both coaching and MI build upon the client-centered approach, employ positive psychology, and assume that people have the inner resources and capability to choose what and how to change. Like MI, life coaching and its numerous subspecialties take a broader view of human growth, focusing on more than transactional change. Both MI and professional coaching empower people to unearth their inner motivations for sustainable change and deeper transformation.

In most cases in this book, we have referred to people in general with plural pronouns, except in specific coaching scenarios where there is one client. The coaching scenarios in this book are compilations of cases that have been disguised and fictionalized. Separately, online you can find reproducible handouts and additional resources for learning and teaching coaching with MI at *www.guilford.com/lanier-materials.*

Acknowledgments

CECILIA LANIER

First, I acknowledge Bill Miller and his cofounder, Stephen Rollnick, for developing motivational interviewing (MI), a person-centered method of helping people change and grow. This book is the result of Bill's vision to offer MI to the world of professional coaching. I am indebted to Bill for his expert mentoring, friendship, and tireless support as the series editor for this book. He believed in me while gently pointing the way forward.

I am also grateful for our author team, Patty Bean and Stacey Arnold. Patty's commitment to details, along with her supportive consultations and discussions, helped to ground the work in authentic coaching practice. Stacey's passion and ability to connect with people were the catalyst for our bravery in embarking on this landmark project. The guidance and experiences of my coaches, mentors, trainees, students, colleagues, and clients continue to teach me and provide lessons on how to respectfully and effectively support people's change and growth. Dr. Ruth Wolever and Leigh-Ann Webster freely offered their expertise in the history, current research, and emerging questions about best practices in coaching.

Finally, I am deeply appreciative of Jim Nageotte, Jane Keislar, and the many other editors at The Guilford Press who balance professionalism with personal kindness in all their careful editing and attention to detail.

PATTY BEAN

I'd like to thank Dr. William Miller for sharing his wisdom and tutelage with the author team. I owe a debt of gratitude to Cecilia for sitting in the chair day after day pounding out the copy—this book would not have happened without her skill, expertise, and perseverance—and to Stacey for her extraordinary research skills. I'm grateful to the International Coaching Federation (ICF) and the National Board of Health and Wellness Coaching (NBHWC) for their efforts to advance the coaching profession and create standards to guide coaches. Thank you to my teachers, past and present; you have taught me to trust my inner wisdom. I so appreciate my former coach students, fellow classmates in my coach-training programs, my coaching mentees, and my coaching clients. You have helped me become the coach I am today. I am grateful for your trust in my abilities. I owe gratitude to my family and friends who have supported and encouraged me on this journey; I love and appreciate you. Lastly, thank you to the Guilford Press editors who have made this book better in every way.

STACEY ARNOLD

I extend my heartfelt gratitude to the following individuals:

Dr. William Miller, for your invaluable insight and unwavering patience in supporting and guiding my writing struggles. Your professionalism, wisdom, and expertise created a friendship I will always cherish.

The Guilford Press and all of the dedicated professionals guiding us through this journey. Thank you for your commitment to quality and for making the entire process an organized and enriching experience.

I sincerely appreciate Cecilia and Patty, whose collaboration, dedication, and commitment to excellence shaped this book.

Ron Arnold, my husband, thank you for your encouragement, insightful feedback, support, and understanding, especially during late nights while I researched.

Mackenzie Donohue, I would like to express my sincere gratitude for your enthusiasm and discerning eye while providing feedback. Thank you.

To my friend Suzie Price, your endless encouragement, kindness, expert advice, and understanding were always a source of comfort. Your friendship is a treasure.

Contents

Purchasers of this book can access a supplementary chapter, "Research on Coaching and Motivational Interviewing"; reproducible handouts for personal use or use with clients; and other training and learning resources at *www.guilford.com/lanier-materials*.

Part I

Coach-Approach Parallels with Motivational Interviewing

Chapter 1

What Is Coaching?

I have ideas and aspirations buried deep inside,
like dying embers. What I need is a matchstick!
—CLIENT

We chose the coaching profession because, at the core, there's nothing quite like witnessing and being a part of a person's journey of growth and change. You, too, may share our passion for making a meaningful difference in people's lives. A personal journey of transformation may have led you here, or maybe you noticed that others lean on and confide in you when they struggle in life or work. Regardless of your unique reason, the resonant heartbeat for all of us is that we believe we have something of profound value to offer people on their path of change and growth.

Many of us have come from other professions. The 2020 International Coaching Federation (ICF) Global Coaching Study reported that 94% of coaches offer services in addition to coaching, such as consulting (60%), training (60%), and/or facilitation services (54%). Coaches are nutritionists, counselors, physical therapists, nurses, yoga instructors, project managers, interior designers, teachers, retired from corporate positions, or a host of other occupations. As fulfilling as those occupations are, we made a shift because we sought something more. Perhaps you wanted to go deeper, become more effective, and see people make lasting change. We decided coaching is the missing piece.

This chapter's central focus is on coaching, and future chapters will build a tight bridge connecting coaching with a conversational approach called motivational interviewing (MI). We make the case that coaching, specifically the practitioner stance referred to as the "coach approach," can be synonymous with MI. MI's principles, method, and spirit can shape the *how* and *what* of our practice and, more importantly, the *why* of our approach. We view MI as foundational for much of the theory, processes, and methods of coaching. The ideas about coaching in this chapter find parallels in MI, which we will fully explore in future chapters.

Whether or not you arrived at coaching from one of the professions named above, you may be aware that a common concept of coaching is that we remove our "expert" hats and instead approach clients as experts in their own lives. You may have experienced receiving a directive, a prescription, or a business plan from an expert in your life, but you did not change. Or maybe you were the expert, and despite your expertise, the person or organization you tried to help made only minimal and short-term adjustments. You can hear the disappointment in this story: A chiropractor shared that he gave a client exercises to strengthen his back, but the client came back and reported that the exercises didn't work. The chiropractor asked, "Did you do them?" The patient replied, "I tried to, but just couldn't get around to it." With a sigh, the chiropractor shook his head regretfully and said, "No, these exercises won't work unless you do them."

Do people need more information and more expertise? Typically, when we need more information, we can just google it. Sometimes more information helps, of course, like knowing what to do to lower our risk of developing cardiovascular disease. But for behavior change, more information alone does not always inspire action. Real change often happens in a relationship between people who engage and connect with each other. This awareness is pervasive in our culture and especially noticeable in work environments. "Organizations have come to understand that effective performance depends on effective relationships" (Kimsey-House et al., 2018, p. xi). You came to coaching not only to find out what to say and do but, more importantly, *how* to say it in a way that ignites the smoldering motivation for change and growth in your clients. The relationship is key. Our experience testifies that speaking louder or adding more information is not the formula for facilitating behavior change. Passion, experience, and various levels of expertise in diverse fields are not enough to make us more effective. We need something else.

Can people simply change on their own? Yes, we all make changes, driven by our desires and hopes for a better existence. We choose a better job, clean out our desk drawer, start drinking more water, or turn in work projects on time. And yet, at times, we may have something in our life that is not budging. Maybe we do not manage our stress, and we eat or drink our emotions or work to exhaustion and neglect our families. Humans are not usually all or nothing when it comes to behavior change but are more beautifully nuanced than that. Herein lies the dilemma of human growth and development. We find that people often want and need to change but find themselves stuck in the current dilemma. As coaches, we can do something to loosen the grip of the status quo and invite clients to declare, "I'm ready!" We can help the self-changers get started and then walk with them on the forward-moving path toward change and growth.

THE COACHING RELATIONSHIP

Coaching is first a relationship. But it is not one of imbalance of roles or status, where one person descends while the other rises high, like children on a seesaw. In coaching, two experts, the coach and the client, form a partnership to benefit the client's self-directed ongoing change and growth. As a coach, you bring your expertise to the relationship. Having the finesse to know when and how to dispense expertise is the skill of a masterful coach. Although we stay in our scope and do not claim to diagnose or cure, we simultaneously stand as developing experts in behavior change.

This balanced partnership calls forth a creative and thoughtful process that inspires clients to reach their highest personal or professional goals, their ideal and authentic selves. In this relationship, clients are engaged, active, learning, discovering, and using self-monitoring to work toward their goals. The coaching relationship focuses energy on empowering clients' self-regulation and self-directed change, which is the end purpose of coaching. Skilled coaches use behavior change theory, which includes strategies in motivation and communication, all of which inspire intrinsic motivation toward lasting change (Wolever et al., 2013).

The priority of the coaching relationship is where we begin to build our definition of coaching. It can be tempting to skip ahead and grab the tools and strategies of coaching, but we choose to percolate here for a bit. Without this foundational relationship, the how-tos and methods will lack context and may become flat. The danger is that you could default back into the role of expert, one who tells, directs, teaches, consults, or counsels your clients. Coaching is unique, and the coaching relationship is one element that makes it so. Relationships are inherently dependent on the individuals within the team, so it makes sense to focus on the personal characteristics that can enhance this relationship. See Chapter 2 for research on the positive effects of this relationship in psychotherapy, and we assert, in coaching as well.

WHAT COACHES BELIEVE

This chapter describes what the coach approach is, which includes how a coach thinks about the people they serve. What we believe often shapes how we show up as a coach and, thus, how we function as a partner in the coaching relationship. Eckhart Tolle says it well: "Doing is never enough if you neglect being." *Being* is something that includes a mindset, which then translates to words and actions. Here we shine a spotlight on the "being" part, your mindset, your beliefs about other people, specifically your assumptions about the client.

When we use the term "coach" in this book, we are referring to professional coaches. Since the emergence of coaching more than 25 years ago, professional coaching definitions have included globally recognized ideas and beliefs about people and how they change. If these ideas are new to you, we invite you to explore how they can positively impact and influence your coaching.

In the coaching relationship, we believe clients are partners, not patients. They want meaningful change and want to achieve their highest potential and become more of what they know they can be. Furthermore, clients are experts in their own lives; they know what is best for themselves. They are resourceful and capable of creating their own goals and solving their own problems. They can be driven by higher values, and they are able to choose what is most important to them (International Coaching Federation, 2022). Additionally, coaching clients on a professional journey have what it takes to create and achieve their personal best and, in turn, contribute a higher value to their organization or project. We hold to the belief that people possess their own inner genius, and coaching can remind them of that.

Effective coaching begins with this fundamental and non-negotiable belief system. This belief system should undergird every process, method, tool, and technique in coaching. Without this approach, coaching could easily default to the typical model described earlier, one of giving directions, protocols, and prescriptions. You might mistake your role as a "fixer" for fragile people who need to be told what to do or as a dispenser of a prescription for flourishing. Your belief that clients are creative, resourceful, and whole establishes the kind of relationship that is the best container for growth (Kimsey-House et al., 2018). We believe every individual deserves to be treated with respect, and they are worthy of high regard despite their current journey or the reasons for being where they are. Our positive regard for them is unconditional (Rogers, C. R., 1980).

You may be saying, "But wait a minute. Some of my clients look like they have plenty of room for improvement; they don't seem whole. Some of them are scattered and in need of help. And if they are so creative, why can't they seem to figure out a way to move forward? If they're resourceful, why do they need a coach? If they are experts on themselves, why are they still stuck in unhealthy behaviors or struggling to find ways to improve, change, and grow? Why is the organization not growing or the leader not leading? Why don't they fix themselves?"

Yes, this paradox demands an even more tenacious grip on your belief system. But you, as a coach, can consciously choose to see beyond the apparent contradictions. You can build robust relationships with your clients within a framework of acceptance, mutual respect, and trust. Your clients need to feel safe and free to discover, experiment, learn, and grow. Anything short of this could sound the alarm for a client to resist, defend, and make a case for the status quo. It seems ironic, of course, but research suggests that when people who want to change are pushed by someone or something else, they most often hold to the safety of the current situation, and at worst, they push back (Miller & Rollnick, 2013). When people feel accused or judged, a typical response is to remain stuck. This applies to parenting; for example, if parents show continual disapproval of their child, rebellion is a common defense response (Seltzer, 2019).

A coach takes a humble, supportive posture in working with clients. You deeply listen with compassion, and partner with the client to guide, support, invite, and elicit their own journey forward. Only with this humility and compassion will you be able to advocate for your clients' wholeness, wherever they are on their journeys. Even when clients are frozen at a crossroads, these beliefs can breathe hope into their lives, enabling them to move forward. Furthermore, when you have and express confidence in your clients, they are more likely to find the courage and self-efficacy to take the next steps toward their goals (Moore et al., 2016).

You may feel a sense of disequilibrium as you step out of an expert role. After all, many of us are trained to bring knowledge and expertise to people. Adopting this heart and mindset is your first goal as a coach, and with intentional focus, this can be further developed. You will likely find more ease in coaching as you learn to stretch those mindset muscles. Below is a list of the beliefs that shape what we do and how we show up to coaching.

What Coaches Believe

- Clients deserve unconditional positive regard.
- Clients are worthy of respect as they are.
- Clients benefit from an ally who elicits and uncovers their ideas and plans for growth.
- Clients deserve your acceptance and esteem, regardless of their current challenges.
- Clients have the potential to live up to the vision of their ideal selves and futures.
- Clients are capable of making their own decisions (and should be encouraged to do so).
- The coach–client relationship exists to benefit your client.
- Clients are the experts in their own lives.
- All change is self-change; you guide self-changers to choose and act on their goals.
- Clients possess their own unique strengths, motivations, and resources.
- A collaborative partnership with your client enhances growth.
- Motivation already exists within your client; it cannot be installed by you, the coach.

- You can empower your clients by evoking and eliciting their own motivation.
- The coaching relationship is a safe container for clients to imagine and plan for growth.

THE COACH'S ROLE

Assuming you have adopted the heart and mindset necessary for effective practice, then what is your role? How does this look in practice? You may wonder, "What good is our expertise if we can't use it? Is it not a disservice if we withhold information? If clients have the answers, then why do they need coaches?" Some clients want to be told what to do, and others may know what to do but have few resources for how to get it done. We will answer these questions with specific strategies in upcoming chapters, but for now we focus our discussion more on *how* we do what we do. This is part of what we mean when we say, "coach approach."

You, as a coach, may possess vast experience and varying degrees of expertise, yet you set aside your own agenda to give space for your clients to explore their own. You may be an expert in many things, but you remove your expert hat in favor of honoring and eliciting your clients' expertise. You may be able to see further down the road than your clients, but you patiently shine a flashlight on their sometimes-dim path, illuminating one step and then another so they can navigate their way forward. In other words, you wait, guide, and partner with clients to develop their own creative solutions. Your role in this partnering relationship is to build trust and respect so clients are inspired to create their own solutions or partner with you to find new ones. Why do coaches do this? The simple answer is that when people generate their own ideas, they are much more likely to find the internal motivation that sparks the trajectory of growth forward (Ryan & Deci, 2000).

Deci and Ryan's (1985) self-determination theory richly confirms this phenomenon. They identified three basic psychological needs that must be met before self-regulation occurs: autonomy, competence, and relatedness. Coaching is a means to an end, and this end is the client's independence and self-regulation in behaviors that support health and well-being in personal and professional growth. Since the support of autonomy in the coaching relationship is vital to fuel motivation, coaches encourage clients to choose behaviors based on their own values and desires, not those chosen for them (Moore et al., 2016). Clients driven by self-regulation and intrinsic motivation develop greater positive outcomes that are long lasting.

The belief system we describe in this chapter spreads a layer of rich and fertile soil. This primed garden plot is the perfect place to plant the seeds of understanding about what coaching is and how to do it in a masterful and effective way. In later chapters, we offer more specific guidelines for the processes, tools, and coaching techniques. For now, the belief system, the way you approach clients and coaching, is primary and foundational; it's the form within which you eventually bloom with your own voice.

THE COACH APPROACH

How does this approach help you coach clients who know full well what should be done, yet waffle and hesitate? Or how does it help you with clients who do not know what to do or where to get started? How does this approach empower clients to find that internal motivation necessary to propel their lives forward?

Coaching is quite different from what doctors do, the so-called medical model. That approach includes diagnosing, prescribing, and treating symptoms. In the medical model patients may hear the reasons for change, how their lives will improve if they change, and how much harm is done by not changing. They might walk away from a medical consult better informed, though often frustrated or bewildered because they cannot or will not change their harmful lifestyle behaviors. It is no surprise this approach has a poor track record of leading to behavior change. Consider a study in the *Journal of the American Medical Association* that reported that only 4.3% of participants who had a cardiac event and were instructed to make lifestyle changes to prevent recurrence actually made any changes (Brinks et al., 2017). The traditional medical model has focused on one factor: providing information. However, it is clear that knowledge alone is not sufficient to help patients improve their health (Shearn, 2001).

What makes coaching so powerful and effective is not what information you offer or topics you address but *how* you approach things. "Health coaches believe clients are already experts in their own lives and their own needs," said Leigh-Ann Webster, executive director of the National Board for Health and Wellness Coaching (Webster, 2020).

If you hold to this belief that clients are experts in their own lives, then you will approach the coaching relationship in a particular way. Although your preferred style or method may be unique and shaped by your own comfort level and skill, an effective coach will be grounded in the conviction that clients know what is best for them.

Experts are indeed necessary in the face of an immediate crisis. Still, preaching or teaching is not the ideal or most effective way when people seek a behavior change—when they want to lose weight, handle stress better, or adopt a positive mindset when dealing with negative employees. Giving someone a diet plan, a strength-training program, or a webinar on positive emotions and stress reduction does not automatically transfer to action and growth.

The *way* you, as a coach, believe, speak, and act is the very thing that sets coaching apart from many typical helper models. As a coach, you take on the privilege and responsibility to stir a person's own expertise and their own inner motivation, and then you walk alongside them to start and sustain change. Again, we know the question may linger for some: "How do you help someone change if you don't tell them what to do?" Propelled by this paradox, excellence in coaching departs from the typical model and adopts the coach approach as a way to be most effective.

Often, clients know what they want but have not found the motivation within themselves to get where they want to go. Coaching can make a difference, says Leigh-Ann Webster. According to Webster, this client-directed approach is key, and as we will explore later, it is based on MI.

> In this technique, health coaches ask non-judgmental, open-ended questions that provide opportunities for clients to explore their motivation for change and, in collaboration with their coach, develop strategies to change their behavior that are personally meaningful and self-directed. (Webster, 2021)

When you, as a coach, hold a particular heart and mindset about your clients, you discover that these beliefs naturally circulate and breathe life into how you treat people. Your beliefs determine your thoughts, and those thoughts determine your behavior and actions. The trade secret is that this, in turn, has a direct impact on your clients' progress. Your beliefs about your clients indirectly influence their growth trajectory toward health and fulfillment in life and work (Moore et al., 2016).

The coach approach calls on clients to become the decision-makers, to grow into discovering (or rediscovering) their own expertise on a path forward. You help by calling forth what is deep inside each client. If you do not believe in the capacity of your clients, it can impede their growth toward health and well-being. Furthermore, holding your clients in high regard is a prerequisite for establishing trust and rapport and building relationships that inspire self-efficacy and confidence in your clients.

These unique views are the life pulse of everyone who calls themselves a coach and embraces the coach approach. You acknowledge that people are capable of finding answers, choosing, taking action, and bouncing back when hitting roadblocks, and, of course, they are capable of learning. In the book *Co-Active Coaching*, the authors asserted this recognition is more than a belief, "It is a stand we take" (Kimsey-House et al., 2018). See Table 1.1 for a comparison of what the coach approach is and is not.

THE HISTORY OF COACHING AND THE COACH APPROACH

To the best of our knowledge, the definition of the term "coach approach" finds its origins in the 1980's field of business consultants. According

TABLE 1.1. The Coach Approach Is, Is Not

The coach approach is . . .

1. Showing support and empathy for your clients.
2. Honoring clients as experts in their own lives.
3. Enabling clients to exercise autonomy.
4. Accepting that clients are creative, resourceful, and whole.
5. Demonstrating positive regard for clients.
6. Forming working alliances to create shared goals that are important to your clients.
7. Personalizing the coaching process for each client's learning and growth.
8. A client-centered, client-driven agenda.
9. Using MI skills (open-ended questions, affirmations, reflections, and summaries) to evoke and empower clients to self-discover motivation to change and grow.
10. Acknowledging and inquiring about your clients' expressed or unexpressed emotions and shifts in energy.
11. Listening deeply to understand your clients, which includes waiting for them to speak.
12. Adopting an attitude and posture of curiosity and humility in service to your clients.
13. A professional growth mindset that is open to ongoing reflection, feedback, and learning from peers, mentors, or clients.
14. Inviting self-awareness and intrinsic motivation by helping clients align their current reality and goals with their larger vision.

The coach approach is not . . .

1. Showing pity or sympathy for your clients.
2. Assuming clients need your expertise.
3. Inserting your expertise in clients' decisions.
4. Believing that clients are broken and may not be able to create ideas and solutions.
5. Demonstrating judgment toward your clients.
6. Forming a coach-driven relationship where you set or suggest goals for your clients.
7. Using a one-size-fits-all protocol without personalization for your clients' needs.
8. A coach-driven agenda.
9. Asking yes/no questions, evaluating, advising, or persuading your clients to become more motivated to change and grow.
10. Overlooking or minimizing your clients' expressed or unexpressed emotions and shifts in energy.
11. Talking more than your clients and filling the empty space with your comments.
12. Assuming that that you already know what your clients want and need to do.
13. A professional fixed mindset that resists feedback, and does not seek input from peers, mentors, or your clients.
14. Overly focusing on your clients' short-term goals and failing to cultivate motivation by connecting to their longer-range visions and goals for their ideal self and future.

to Michael Arloski, author of *Wellness Coaching for Lasting Lifestyle Change* and CEO of Real Balance Global Wellness Services, Inc. (*www.realbalance.com*), the term "coach approach" is synonymous with the origins of professional coaching itself. In the 1980s, some business consultants began to expand their services beyond providing in-depth analysis and strategic planning. They included teaching supportive relationship skills such as listening, establishing accountability, and helping clients set up goals and plans to finally achieve "whatever had been eluding them" (M. Arloski, personal communication, August 5, 2021).

One of the earliest pioneers in the field was Thomas Leonard, along with the authors of *Co-Active Coaching*, Henry and Karen Kimsey-House, Phil Sandahl, and Laura Whitworth (2018). From this group, the definition and practice of coaching took shape. Their work led to the formation of the International Coaching Federation (ICF) in 1995 and then the ICF core coaching competencies. (The ICF core coaching competencies are available online. We have created a link to them at *www.guilford.com/lanier-materials.*). These competencies drew a framework around coaching characteristics as distinct from consulting (Dueease, 2009).

According to Dueease, Leonard and Kimsey-House applied their business backgrounds and created what we now call coaching. Leonard invented "personal coaching" and was responsible for the coach training curriculum for Coach U and then, afterward, the Coach Training Institute. He designed the personal coaching process.

Life coaching was popularized in the early 2000s with the explosion of "reality" shows where many self-proclaimed life coaches involved themselves in the personal lives of others. But it was Thomas Leonard who dubbed this uniquely developed process "personal coaching" because it assists people by focusing on the inner person. Leonard's newly created process filled a blank spot among the other existing human improvement processes. A recent study by the *Harvard Business Review* confirmed Leonard's perspective that all coaching focuses on personal issues. The study of 140 executive coaches reported that while only 3% of coaches were *hired* to assist in the personal lives of executives, over 75% of coaches found that they actually were helping their clients with personal issues (Dueease, 2009).

For this reason, when we speak of coaching in this book, we refer broadly to the field of life coaching, which includes certain subspecialties, such as health and wellness coaching.

A Working Definition of the Coach Approach

While in coach training, we heard the term "coach approach" many times, but as we began to write this book, we could not find a succinct definition that described the uniqueness of this approach we wanted to convey. This quest for a clear definition of the coach approach was the inspiration for this chapter.

While some attempts to define the coach approach include a list of strategies and skills, we humbly assert that many definitions omit the more important fundamental element of the coach's belief system. Here's our definition of the coach approach, as explained in this chapter:

> *The coach approach is a unique set of foundational beliefs and behaviors that shape the coaching conversations to inspire client-initiated consideration and plans for growth and change. The beliefs and behaviors, based on evidence-based change theories, form a container for a relationship that empowers clients as autonomous experts in their lives. Clients have resources, capabilities, and ideas for discovering why, how, and what to do to achieve their desires and goals. The relationship is built on compassion for people, acceptance of who they are and their situation, partnering with them to support their goals, and empowering them to find their motivations for change and growth.*

(See Handout 1.1 at *www.guilford.com/lanier-materials* for an extended definition.)

Some may mistake coaching as a means of giving advice or information, figuratively blowing an air horn on a person's bad behavior or giving out awards and incentives for a job well done. But as we have discussed already, people do not make changes because an expert tells them to do something or praises them for their behavior. Effective coaching is much more than a way to mentor, train, teach, consult, advise, or counsel people. While those methods have merit in the proper context, they are not suited for the partnering-style relationship found in coaching.

As a coach, you do not diagnose, prescribe, or claim to cure. You do not threaten, cajole, warn, or even reward behavior to get people to change. Yet neither do you passively listen and nod in agreement or sympathy. Instead, you skillfully and dynamically navigate a collaborative relationship that invites and inspires your client's growth.

A STANDARD OF PRACTICE: OUR COMPASS

As a coach, you hardly need convincing that coaching works. You are here because you know coaching is a powerful intervention for people who want to change. But as we pivot our focus to standards, core competencies, and credentialing, it may be worth reminding ourselves why these are so important in this field.

Clients expect and deserve a consistent quality and predictable service across a broad range of coaching contexts. According to the 2020 ICF

Global Coaching Study, most managers/leaders who use coaching skills agree that clients expect their coaches to be certified or credentialed. The number of respondents who agreed rose from 37% in 2015 to 55% in 2019 (ICF, 2020b). Clients expect a level of proficiency and skill when employing a coach. In this case, becoming credentialed and meeting proficiency standards is simply a matter of rising to the level of expectations of those you hope to serve.

National standards and international core competencies assure clients and the public that certified or credentialed coaches throughout the field possess a core base of knowledge and skills and a certain level of proficiency. Clients who join with a coach who received national or international recognition as a competent coach can be reassured that they receive the best available service, regardless of their location.

THE CASE FOR STANDARDS, CORE COMPETENCIES, AND CREDENTIALS

These days, coaches are expected to be competent and credentialed, especially when a client makes a significant investment in coaching. An article in *Forbes Coaches Council* (Young, 2021) spells out what consumers (specifically, business executives) should look for when hiring a coach.

In that article the author outlines some critical characteristics of good coaches and evidence of their expertise in the field, both of which apply to this discussion. First, good coaches use evidence-based methodologies. Second, good coaches are able to customize a plan to fit their clients and get beneath the surface to their clients' deeper needs. Good coaches will be adept at using various techniques and models to suit their clients' unique needs. This customization helps emphasize clients' autonomy, self-confidence, and an accountability plan. Good coaches are able to support clients to connect their goals to a larger vision and greater purpose for their lives.

Finally, credentialed and qualified coaches are happy to verify and authenticate their training, including the program they attended and how many coaching hours were required to complete it. These coaches ideally provide certification from an organization such as the International Coaching Federation (ICF) or board certification from an organization such as the National Board for Health and Wellness Coaching (NBHWC).

Standards are not just for the benefit of the client. They are also for sponsors who depend upon coach services to produce specific outcomes, such as employers, human resources (HR) managers, organization leaders, superintendents, parents, or practitioners in medical practice. These sponsors, or third-party members, focus on the investment and the expected specific outcomes. Whether a coach's client is an individual or an organization, the client increasingly demands a level of service commensurate with the investment of resources. In addition to the benefit to clients and those who employ coaches in their organizations, standards offer many advantages for coaches.

Standards and Competencies: A Path to Professional Integrity

While relaxing around a fire pit, a marketing expert sat across from a new coach, chatting about what messages would be essential to convey on an upcoming website. This marketing expert brazenly demanded, "Don't use the word 'coach' in your branding materials. The modern consumer is tired of the term, and it's been overused and watered-down." Her rationale was based on market research citing how that term was used too broadly. The term could include a range of people: on one end of the continuum those who received no training or attended a weekend seminar and on the other end those who graduated with certification from an accredited program. The public was too savvy, she said, to take this term seriously, and they had become suspicious of what they perceived to be a self-designated title. The coach was stunned at this news.

What do we, as coaches, do with this information? Instead of diminishing and bowing our heads in apology and acquiescence, we can choose to reclaim the term and instead bring it to the rightful and respectable place it deserves in the world of professional services. We can honor the calling and the altruistic model of coaching. Although silence in the coaching conversation is often used to benefit the client, we are certainly not mute in professional integrity. We can speak up and insist that this profession is among the most honorable, fulfilling, and impactful vocations within the personal and professional development professions.

As suggested in the *Forbes Coaches Council* article (Young, 2021), one way to use our voices is to consider becoming nationally board certified by the NBHWC or credentialed through an organization such as the ICF. Many of the concepts in this book are predicated on this assumption: The standards and core competencies are the framework within which we build our professional, ethical, and effective practice. Within these guardrails, we can offer a high-quality service for our clients.

The standards and core competencies are the links that unite coaches in strength and identity. Why are they so central to our identities? They keep us in our lane, within our scope of practice. Standards and core competencies are our compass to keep us traveling in the right direction.

How the Standards Help Us in Coaching

Coaching conversations are a lot like diving off a high dive. The diving skill is only tested once divers take the lonely walk up the ladder and gingerly place their toes right to the edge of the slowly pulsing board. The final movements are fluid and natural. The diver positions themselves, bouncing with precision, until finally, with one last thrust of commitment, they spring high up into the air and take the inevitable descent to the water. It's too late to check the manual of instructions. The momentum takes over, and there is no turning back. The dive is assessed for quality not during the dive but *after* the diver is in the water. You, too, as a coach, enter the coaching session with a commitment, and once it begins, you will focus entirely on the client and the process at hand. You cannot check the list of "most powerful questions," and your notes are out of reach. It's only afterward that you look back and reflect on the quality. How can you learn and grow without stopping and checking your notes during a session? The answer is to, like a diver, build muscle memory. Notice how high divers take themselves through a dive simulation beforehand. You may see them, on the ground, micro move as if they are going through each step, each contortion. Their knowledge and skills are so deeply embedded that they can practice and improve them just by using their imaginations.

Our suggestion is to build a strong base of knowledge and skills to draw from. Choose core competencies and standards from the NBHWC or the ICF and study, revisit, and review them so that they are engrained in your memory. Becoming certified and credentialed will help you increase the possibility that you will be able to rely on muscle memory and provide what is best for each client in the moment.

A summary of the standards and core competencies developed by these two organizations gives us context. This is our mooring. Each set of standards and competencies resonates with the same basic foundational principles and beliefs we embrace and have detailed in this chapter. These may help the developing coach become better grounded in the *why* of the methods and strategies used in coaching sessions, which we will explore in later chapters. For both aspiring and experienced coaches, reviewing these standards will help set the stage for our focus on coaching throughout the remainder of the book. (The NBHWC competencies and the ICF core competencies are available online. We have created a link to them at *www.guilford.com/lanier-materials.*)

You may be tempted to skip ahead and collect the strategies, tips, and tricks of coaching in Parts II and III of this book. But experience tells us that when helping clients with complicated challenges or clients who do not move forward, or even if you are hoping to avoid a potential numbing monotony of overly familiar routines, you would be wise to step back and ask yourself *why* you are doing what you are doing. Ultimately, coaching is about your client's growth, so the question should be "How can I be more effective as a coach?" As we have said rather boldly, your client's growth is partially (if not totally) dependent on your effectiveness as a coach. We believe the coach approach is what makes us effective. The absence of that approach will, at best, minimize your impact, and at worst, it may allow your client to linger in the status quo.

Atul Gawande, in his address to Harvard students at the School of Education on the importance of coaching (Harvard Graduate School of Education, 2012), spoke about the proven correlation between students' growth and the skill of the helping professional appointed to them. The George W. Bush Institute study showed that the most critical determinant in student achievement is not student socioeconomic status, district resources, the leadership of the school, or the use of consistent, systemwide protocols. The one factor that makes the difference is the teacher's level of skill (Goldhaber et al., 2015). Gawande draws a close parallel for coaches. The most important player is not the protocol (strategy or method) but the coach. Therefore, the coach's responsibility is to continue striving for professional growth and mastery of the fundamental concepts of coaching.

Concepts in this first chapter help to steady the footing of the novice, developing, or experienced coach in the *why* of the methods and strategies in coaching. We hope you continue your ongoing journey toward becoming a more effective coach by taking an in-depth review of the coach approach while also continuing your mastery of the core competencies and standards in the field. Next, we venture into the coaching competencies to highlight how the coach approach is integrated throughout our professional standards.

PROFESSIONAL STANDARDS AND COMPETENCIES FOR COACHING

International Coaching Federation

The ICF core competencies were first created in 1998. These provided a vital and early foundation for the coaching profession and set the standard for ethics and practice in the coaching field. The founders sought to define and enlarge the understanding of the skills and knowledge needed for effective coaching.

The updated core competency model has new elements and themes that broaden the existing foundation, including a focus on ethical behavior and confidentiality, the coach's mindset, ongoing reflective practice, coaching agreements, the partnership of the coach and client, and the influence of context and culture on self and others. All eight core competencies can be accessed at the ICF's website (we have provided a link to those competencies at *www.guilford.com/lanier-materials*). In this summary, notice the themes of the coach approach that we have described in this chapter.

1. Ethics and standards of coaching set the foundation for all coaching practice.
2. Coaches develop their own mindset, which is open, curious, flexible, and client centered. Coaches know that clients are responsible for their own choices, just as coaches are responsible for their own emotions, reflective practice, and ongoing learning.
3. Coaches partner with the client and stakeholders to create agreements about the relationship, the overall coaching arrangement, and each individual coaching session.
4. Coaches partner with the client and create a supportive environment that allows clients to feel safe and free to share. The relationship is built on mutual respect and trust.
5. Coaches are fully present with the client, being fully conscious with an open, grounded, flexible, and confident style.
6. Coaches focus on the full meaning of clients' spoken or unspoken communication and further support client self-expression.
7. The coach uses tools and techniques such as questioning, silence, metaphor, or analogy to facilitate client insight and learning.
8. The coach promotes client autonomy by partnering with the client to transform learning and insight into action.

The National Board for Health and Wellness Coaching

The NBHWC was formed in 2012 to advance the profession of health and wellness coaching. In 2016, it collaborated with the National Board of Medical Examiners (*nbme.org*) to create a robust board certification exam, leading to more than 9,400 national board certified health and wellness coaches (NBC-HWC) who hold the credential.

A content outline was created and is now the national board certification examination framework for coaching. Training programs that wish to become approved NBHWC programs adhere to the content outline for the training and education standards. (See the content outline at NBHWC's website; we have provided a link to that website at *www.guilford.com/lanier-materials*). Instead of summarizing the 126 competencies and related skills, we present the beautifully succinct yet comprehensive definition of coaching stated in the NBHWC code of ethics:

> Health and Wellness coaches partner with clients seeking self-directed, lasting changes aligned with their values, which promote health and wellness and, thereby, enhance well-being. In the course of their work, health and wellness coaches display unconditional positive regard for their clients and a belief in their capacity for change and honoring that each client is an expert on his or her life while ensuring that all interactions are respectful and non-judgmental. (NBHWC, 2017)

The ICF and NBHWC competencies echo the coach approach described in this chapter. One can see why these standards are considered essential and foundational to the practice of all coaches in all fields.

In the chapters to come, we will make the case that this coach approach, along with the competencies and standards, receives direction and inspiration from the theory and practice of MI. As you continue in this book, you will hear MI as the unmistakable melody that harmonizes with all discussions of coaching theories, models, methods, and techniques.

COACH-APPROACH SAMPLE

This short coaching scenario is an example of how a coach can use the coach approach. Here, we spotlight a few applications of the ICF core competencies and the coach approach.

John arrives for his second coaching session. In the beginning and after reviewing how things have gone for him since the last session, the coach elicits John's focus for this session. She frames her responses around the belief that John has the answers he needs within himself, and she resists stepping into a fix-it, expert mode. She is self-aware and consciously decides to hold a nonjudgmental belief in the client's value, worth, and potential. (CA, coach approach; ICF, International Coaching Federation core competencies.)

COACH: You wanted to work on getting fit. What specifically do you want to accomplish in our time together?	CA: *Client-led agenda, honoring autonomy.* ICF 3.6: Partners to identify what clients want to accomplish in the session.
CLIENT: I can't get myself motivated or in that mindset where, "Okay, I'm going to do this." My wife and I already eat healthy food, but I need to get strong and fit for my health and be an example for my boys. I'm not where I want to be right now.	
COACH: It's important to you, because you want to feel strong and be an example. That's the bottom line: You recognize that something's missing in your mindset. (*Pause*)	CA: *Expresses empathy, without judgment. Reflects possible meaning, seeking to understand. Coach honors client's autonomy.*

COACH: So, what would make this session of value to you?	ICF 3.8: Partners to define measures of success for the individual session.
CLIENT: I want a plan on paper to look at each day, a plan for food, hydration, and workout so I can be focused. Mental notes aren't working.	
COACH: A paper plan would help you focus. What else needs to be addressed?	CA: *Honors client choice and autonomy.*
CLIENT: I don't really know where to start. What do you think might work for me?	
COACH: Sure, we can dive into that today. What are some ways you've created success in the past around getting fit, building muscle, and losing weight?	CA: *Restrains from the expert role to call on the client's own resources for success.*
CLIENT: The healthiest I've felt and looked was when I was on the paleo food plan, but I was also weightlifting. I'm too busy to go to the gym, and I don't like running. I need something fun, something right for me, maybe weightlifting.	
COACH: You have self-awareness about what works for you, and you want something fun, that gives you results. What would it look like to "spice it up"?	CA: *Sees client as resourceful, and capable of finding solutions. Coach reflects to demonstrate empathy.*

Part of the appeal of this coach approach is born from experience as a teacher. I (C. H. L.) found a new way that aligns with MI to approach students and their learning process.

THE COACH APPROACH: A PERSONAL JOURNEY

As a former teacher, I developed a method for creating a room full of independent learners, in part because I followed the advice, "You can get anything done, as long as you don't mind who gets the credit." My secret was getting students to develop their own ideas, rules, rewards, and most importantly, their *why* for learning. For several years prior to that, I followed the typical model of creating rules and boundaries in hopes of getting students to comply.

If you fail to manage student behavior, the likelihood that you can teach them is low. I used colorful, motivational checklists and incentives to reinforce good behavior and squelch the bad. When students took their behavior reports home, I expected their parents to sort things out and send kids back on Monday morning more well-behaved and ready to comply. But this didn't work! The more resistant kids were no less resistant on Monday morning.

The "meaningful" consequences I set up worked, but only temporarily. The moment I turned away, they went right back to their rascally ways. I noticed a pattern developing, so I took a bird's eye view and asked, "What do I really want for these students?" I wanted them to *want* to learn, be excited, and become independent and self-directed in learning. I knew that was a big ask, but as I went after it with vigor, that success became a pivotal moment in my profession. For the remainder of my teaching career, I enjoyed mostly independent, self-motivated, energized learners in my class. These were not the "easy kids." My reputation for being effective with the more challenging students placed an imaginary sign over my door that said, "Bring me all the hardest cases! I'll spark their love of learning!" And that is exactly what happened.

How did I do this? First, I shifted my mindset. Instead of demanding respect from students, I began with the notion that they deserved respect and unconditional positive regard. I was trained in a behavioral management technique whose approach was built around the work of Carl Rogers, who developed the idea that a person should be accepted and respected as they are, without judgment (Rogers, 1951). With a new mindset, everything changed. I no longer viewed some students as apathetic, incompetent, or misbehaved, and more profoundly, I stopped treating them that way. How did this belief transform students into energized and self-motivated learners?

My new beliefs changed my approach. Tossing out the charts and checklists, I met the students as partners, asking them what and how they wanted to learn (while staying within the mandated curriculum standards). I honored their ideas and encouraged their involvement and creativity, and was thrilled and even surprised at how many ideas they had and how excited they were to learn and exert their autonomy. The positive results confirmed the power of this approach. Once I stopped overtelling and overdirecting them and invited them alongside the learning journey, they took off! Soon, my classroom became an observation point for university-level intern teachers looking for models of effective instruction. Interns, with clipboards ready, wanted to know tips and tricks and best-practice strategies: the secrets. Strategies are helpful, but I insisted they have minimal impact if you neglect the foundation, the thinking and believing part.

Years later, I transitioned to the role of instructional coach for teachers and witnessed—again—the power of my beliefs to influence my words and actions and, ultimately, the teacher's ownership and investment in their own growth. I watched teachers whose once sparkling enthusiasm had been dulled by the increasingly high demands of the job. Some were frustrated and felt trapped in the status quo. How would I engage these dedicated professionals to choose goals for improvement? How could I spark their first love to create ideas and help them set new goals for becoming more effective instructors? How would I elicit the excitement and energy necessary to make changes, even while they were already spinning many plates on the job?

As I did with the students, I began with respect and unconditional positive regard. I believed in the teachers' capability even though they might sit in a meeting with folded arms, shrugging their shoulders when asked for a plan. I met them as equal partners in this relationship of mutual trust and communicated my message loud and clear. I respected them as experts in their own practice. Since our district's directive was to make my program entirely voluntary, I had to wait for them to choose coaching. They would never have invited me in if they had any hint that our coaching meetings would result in more demands, criticism, or judgment.

Soon, they believed I was there to support them, and eventually, they also asked for my advice and suggestions. But I waited to be asked. Instead of scrutinizing their practice, I demonstrated compassion and empathy and supported their self-created goals with reflective discussion. As cited in a districtwide review of the coaching initiative, the success of this approach proved the validity and benefits of coaching. Growth ignited! The coach approach unlocked their inner genius or, rather, helped them rediscover it.

One surprising bonus was that they began working within professional learning teams. And in this case, teamwork proved to be equally if not more impactful than one-on-one sessions. This changed the culture of professional learning and instruction in the school and, as a result, had a positive data-proven impact on student achievement. The district was more than pleased with the investment in coaching.

This narrative illustrates how heart and mindset (fundamentals of the coach approach) are a starting point for effective helping. Professional coaching is framed within the same paradigm. A coach is a partner who respects the client's abilities, values, and reasons as valid and sufficient for meaningful change and growth. The coach approach is the vital foundation that allows this to happen.

Take It Further

Directions: Work with a partner or in your professional learning community to read and follow the instructions and respond to each of the questions below.

1. Find the NBHWC competencies that focus on building the coaching partnership, including the client's self-discovery and the coach's role in the relationship. (We have put a link to these competencies at *www.guilford.com/lanier-materials.*)
   a. Identify the statements that are descriptive of the coach approach.
   b. In your own words, write out the coach's primary function.
2. Find the NBHWC competencies that focus on establishing trust and rapport in the coaching relationship.
   a. Describe the benefits gained by establishing trust and rapport.
3. Find the NBHWC competencies that focus on the client's freedom of choice, autonomy, and intrinsic motivation.
   a. What does this say about eliciting and evoking a client's motivation?
4. Find an ICF and an NBHWC core competency supporting the idea that the coach is not the expert. Explain why this is important in coaching.
5. Locate the Handout 1.1 online at *www.guilford.com/lanier-materials.* Read the four sections that define the coach approach. Work in your learning community to discuss ways in which this approach is similar to or different from your own experiences and ideas.

Chapter 2

Evidence for Coaching with Motivational Interviewing

How well does coaching work, and what about coaching with MI? What difference does using the coach approach make in the final outcome? If coaching is effective, what components have been shown to make a successful outcome more likely? We are thrilled that the field of coaching is interested in researching and clarifying coaching's effectiveness and answering these questions. Our discussion of the relationship component of the coach approach in Chapter 1 is a good place to begin the search.

MI sets the bar high with a commitment to using scientific methods to test what works, and this chapter provides a broad summary of those findings to date. For coaching, we review early evidence that points to the coach–client relationship as a pivotal factor for success. We also examine the current research on the effectiveness of coaching, the evidence base for MI, and the effectiveness of coaching with MI.

COACHING AS AN EVIDENCE-INFORMED METHOD

The coaching profession strives to ground its work in evidence-informed practices, similar to other helping professions. This is especially important because coach licensure is not currently required in the United States. A variety of coach training programs exist with differences in length, depth, and scope; some are weekend workshops, and others require a 2-year commitment. Several colleges and universities offer coach training as part of their curriculum. Regardless of our training, we coaches can distinguish ourselves and our profession by incorporating evidence-based methods such as MI.

The Coaching Relationship as a Key to Effectiveness

A task-force analysis of evidence-based therapy relationships related the quality of the relationship to the effectiveness of therapy. This review of the therapeutic relationship concluded that clients improve (or fail to improve) as a result of the therapy relationship as much as the particular treatment method (Norcross & Wampold, 2011). That statement deserves emphasis; the relationship between therapist and client accounts for success as much as does the methods or techniques used. Another investigation confirmed that the therapeutic working alliance is the best predictor of psychotherapy outcomes (Safran et al., 1990; Luborsky et al., 1983).

Although those studies review therapeutic relationships in psychotherapy, we believe it is reasonable to consider applying this conclusion to the client–coach relationship. Later, we review research that makes the case that the quality of the client–coach relationship is the best predictor of client success. Furthermore, as we said in Chapter 1, we assert that a coach's attitudes and beliefs shape or provide the possibility for a high-quality relationship, which in turn allows a client to make and sustain change.

Results of an investigation with 30 coach–client pairs found that the quality of the coaching relationship predicted the coaching outcome. The characteristics of a quality relationship include client self-efficacy, confidence, independence, and competence in adopting and maintaining change behavior (Baron & Morin, 2012). But what coach qualities are shown to be most helpful?

One study found that clients value a coach's relationship skills, such as empathic listening, understanding, and positive encouragement (de Haan et al., 2011). Another study discovered that rapport, connection, and the perception of a caring coach relationship were vital components in the successful transition from hospitalization to self-managed home care (Parry et al., 2006).

Qualitative research followed six coaches and nine participant clients who received integrated health coaching sessions by telephone. The clients reported the value of the supportive relationship with the health coach. They also took an active role in achieving their self-defined goals and increasing mindfulness to affect change, and reported a sense of personal health and well-being transformation. They took ownership of and responsibility for their goals and reported changes in mental and physical health, including increased exercise and self-care activities, improved nutrition, and additional lifestyle modifications. The participants also reported changes at work, in their relationships at home and at work, and in their personal development (Goble et al., 2017).

The Common Thread between Coaching and Therapy

Although coaching and therapy overlap in some ways, their purposes differ. Coaching facilitates clients' movement from a neutral point (or average performance) toward a more ideal and optimal level of functioning. Therapy treats patients who are functioning below their normal and moves them toward the absence of illness, disease, or low functioning. Patients seeking therapy may be functioning below average and seek help to get back to normal (De Haan, 2011).

Against the backdrop of the discussion of the coach approach in Chapter 1, we highlight one significant parallel between coaching and therapy: the importance of the relationship. The book *Effective Psychotherapists* (Miller & Moyers, 2021) emphasizes the positive impact that an effective relationship can have on client success. The key components of this therapeutic relationship include accurate empathy, acceptance, positive regard, genuineness, focus, hope and expectation, evoking, and offering information and advice. Empathy involves deep listening to understand the client's perspective instead of listening to formulate a reply. Those relational components and skills are further explored in Chapter 4.

The central role of these relational components is echoed in the ICF and the NBHWC coaching competencies and skills guidelines.

Supportive Relationship in the ICF Competencies

The ICF competencies promote a supportive relationship built on the foundation of trust and safety.

> ICF Competency B.4—Co-Creating the Relationship: Cultivates Trust and Safety
> ICF B.4.1—Seeks to understand the client within their context which may include their identity, environment, experiences, values and beliefs.
> ICF B.4.2.—Demonstrates respect for the client's identity, perceptions, style and language and adapts one's coaching to the client.
> ICF B.4.3—Acknowledges and respects the client's unique talents, insights, and work in the coaching process.
> ICF B.4.4—Shows support, empathy and concern for the client.

(The ICF Core Competencies [2019] are used with permission from the ICF. The ICF Core Competencies can be accessed at *https://coachingfederation.org/credentials-and-standards/core-competencies*.)

Supportive Relationship in the NBHWC Competencies

Likewise, the NBHWC competencies also promote a supportive relationship built on the foundation of trust and rapport. (Refer to the NBHWC materials available via the website: *www.guilford.com/lanier-materials*.) Within a positive environment where they feel accepted, clients are more apt to be honest and explore their values and internal motivation. In this relationship, your confidence in the client's ability to grow and gain insight is an important ingredient for supporting their self-efficacy. The competencies highlight how you can build trust by noticing not only words and actions but your clients' emotions as well. This may mean that if you sense conflict or confusion, you will acknowledge this with your curious interest.

Some of the key components of an effective therapeutic relationship named above, such as accurate empathy, acceptance, positive regard, genuineness, hope, and expectation, are parallel to the NBHWC coaching competencies. These competencies call on you to embrace authenticity, kindness, sincerity, and honesty. Your unconditional positive regard for your clients will be evident in the way you coach. For example, you will follow through on commitments made to your clients, and if necessary, you will address any potential discord or conflict and seek to resolve it quickly. Additionally, the competencies highlight the advantages of building a trusting environment. Your clients will feel safe to try out new ideas and behaviors, and you will help them develop a growth mindset—one that views growth as a series of experiments and continued efforts.

Empathy and Rapport in the NBHWC Competencies

Accurate empathy can be seen as your attempt to understand your clients' thoughts, perspectives, or emotional state. The related NBHWC competencies describe how you will reflect with empathy and non-judgmental, supportive statements to demonstrate your unconditional positive regard for your clients.

Other related NBHWC competencies also spotlight the importance of trust, respect, and empathy in this safe, supportive relationship. This relationship is foundational and is one that honors your clients' beliefs, perspectives, and emotions. (See Chapter 8 for more on the coach–client relationship.)

Measuring Coaching Effectiveness

In the absence of standardized, objective measures for end-of-session or end-of-term evaluation and feedback, we have a hunch that, like us, you have ways of determining when your coaching is effective. We developed a short list of tools for evaluating and reporting our coaching outcomes, and although some of these are anecdotal and somewhat subjective, they serve a useful function. These types of assessments can both confirm our current approach and signal if and how we might adjust to best fit the client's needs. (See Handout 2.1 at *www.guilford.com/lanier-materials*. Refer to the "Take It Further" section at the end of the chapter for more on how you might use these tools.)

Beyond these self-reports of coaching effectiveness, empirical research supports the critical role of the coach–client relationship for coaching success (Page & de Haan, 2014). In fact, Page and de Haan confirmed that the strength of the coach–client relationship (or working alliance) was the most powerful predictor of coaching outcomes. Your experience may also have confirmed that spending time building a strong relationship with a client becomes the critical component for a successful coaching experience, and this is perceived by both you and the client.

The Need for Evidence of Coaching Effectiveness

Coaching as a discipline is fairly new, and yet there are numerous books, courses, training programs, and undergraduate and graduate master's programs on the topic. Why are so many consultants, therapists, and others interested in becoming coaches? And why do we see professional coaching accreditation groups and international foundations and conferences? According to Page and de Haan (2014), the way coaching is now viewed is one of the reasons for these professional groups. Formerly, coaching was seen as remedial; a coach would fix your problem. Coaching signaled that something was wrong. Now, if a company hires a coach, it signals that the organization is on an upward trajectory of continual improvement. The people within an organization that hires a coach also now often acknowledge that they desire to understand themselves and grow and flourish in the work environment. It's a badge of honor for leaders to admit they had coaching and that they are developing emotional intelligence and vision.

The global coaching profession is becoming more developed and regulated. The 2020 ICF Global Coaching Study reported that the number of professional coach practitioners was estimated to be 71,000, a 33% increase from 2015. A 2004 *Harvard Business Review* article stated that business coaching was a $1 billion industry in the United States and a $2 billion industry worldwide (Sherman & Freas, 2004). Growing pains in the coaching profession suggest that more scrutiny will be critical in validating its effectiveness. Even still, investigation is underway to document the overall outcomes of coaching. Solid studies are needed to show evidence of the effectiveness of coaching and invite constructive examination to help improve and validate the coaching profession.

Benefits for Executive Coaching

Smither et al. (2003), as reported in *The Psychologist* article titled "Does Executive Coaching Work?" (Page & de Haan, 2014), conducted one of the most extensive impact examinations of executive coaching, including

1,202 senior managers tracked over 2 consecutive years. They reported that managers who worked with a coach had more positive feedback from their supervisors, peers, subordinates, and independent researchers.

On a smaller scale, randomized controlled trials have also used self-scoring instead of independent outcome scales. Executive coaching significantly enhanced goal attainment, resilience, and workplace well-being and lowered depression and stress in health care managers compared to the control group (Smither et al., 2003). Similar positive findings were reported in high school teachers who received coaching compared to a control group. Theeboom et al. (2014) found that executive coaching positively impacted performance, well-being, coping, work attitudes, and goal-directed self-regulation. These studies have affirmed that coaching can be an effective intervention for personal and professional growth.

Benefits of Health and Wellness Coaching

In addition to executive coaching, the field of health and wellness coaching has collected a growing body of evidence documenting the positive outcomes of coaching. Thirteen randomized controlled trials have begun to set the field of coaching apart and invite the medical community to take notice. Numerous other qualitative reports, case studies, project demonstrations, and articles have appeared on the scene to record the benefits of coaching by comparing the coach approach to a control group. Early results point to health and wellness coaching as a potentially significant supplement to traditional care for managing blood sugar, diabetes, cancer pain and survival, asthma, and weight loss and for increasing physical activity (Frates et al., 2011). Vale and colleagues reported on 792 cardiac disease patients, and those who received coaching as part of their intervention dropped cholesterol by 21 points (in comparison to a 7-point drop for those who received treatment as usual; Vale et al., 2003).

Another controlled trial (Wolever et al., 2010) looked at the coached group versus the control group for type 2 diabetes, a condition labeled as an epidemic in the United States, where just over one in ten have diabetes, and one in three have prediabetes (Centers for Disease Control and Prevention, 2020b). With these alarming numbers, more effective interventions are necessary, and this trial pointed to coaching as a viable choice for intervention. The remarkable outcome showed that those who received coaching had a significant reduction in their hemoglobin A1c compared to the control group (Wolever et al., 2010).

Chronic conditions like obesity, hypertension, and diabetes are at an all-time high in the United States. Despite the medical costs and loss of quality of life these conditions incur, many people remain in poor health and with destructive lifestyle behaviors. One of the most underused remedies for these conditions is behavior change with dietary and physical activity interventions. And yet, as we highlighted earlier, knowing what to do does not always translate to taking action. This is where health coaches are needed (Rankins, 2016).

Health coaching works, according to a systematic literature review on the impacts of health coaching. This review concluded that coaching leads to statistically significant improvements in weight management, physical activity, and physical and mental health, all of which will impact chronic illness (Yang et al., 2020).

A systematic review and meta-analysis of coaching research for patients with chronic illness showed that health and wellness coaching improved short-term self-efficacy, quality of life, and depressive symptoms (Boehmer et al., 2023).

WHY AND HOW PEOPLE CHANGE

So far, the growing body of evidence confirms that coaching can be effective and that the coach–client relationship is a key factor for success. What additional evidence-based theories and methods might we need to help our clients create lasting change? A basic understanding of change science, including self-determination theory, the transtheoretical model of change, and MI is necessary. We briefly review the first two in this chapter and take a deep dive into MI throughout the rest of this book.

What is necessary to make a lasting behavior change? Is it enough for people to know what they need and then create a tidy list of pros and cons for changing? Will even a moderate degree of desire be enough to prompt a lasting change?

> "I really want to be healthy. If I am, I can keep working and contribute to my family income. I have so much I want to do with my life, and I don't want to miss out because of diabetes. But I've tried for several years, and I just can't seem to make the changes I want to make."

Self-Determination Theory

What makes some people seemingly glide into change while others spiral around the same arguments and never seem to budge? Deci and Ryan (1985), with the self-determination theory, provided insight into this question and explained the conditions under which people make lasting changes. Self-determination theory (SDT) describes motivation along a continuum, ranging from not ready to very ready. Those on the lower end of ready may come to coaching with a referral from a sponsor or a third party. In contrast, people on the more ready end may have identified internal reasons for change, such as their health or a feeling of accomplishment and life purpose. People who make changes for internal reasons apply more effort and feel more satisfied longer than those who do it for external reasons. The more people buy in and own the reasons for change, the more likely they are to succeed.

MI practice is influenced by SDT, which focuses on increasing internal motivation for change by addressing three basic needs: autonomy, competence, and relatedness. As we have discussed, MI coaches build clients' autonomy by paying careful attention to the partnership and allowing clients to act as capable agents of their own lives.

Competence is the belief in one's ability to change a specific behavior. To succeed, your clients need to believe the change is both important and attainable. You build their competence by encouraging your clients to work on their chosen goals, those that are important to them. You further develop their competence by focusing on what is right with them, spotting and affirming their strengths and efforts.

The power of relatedness is often an underappreciated but important aspect of change, since change is more likely when people are supported by those within their social circle. People will engage in behaviors that are considered meaningful to them and to others with whom they associate. Relatedness also includes the relationship between you and the client. As mentioned, this relationship plays a crucial role in client outcomes.

An important finding from more than 1,000 research studies concluded that the amount of change attributable to the therapeutic relationship is about seven times more than is attributable to a specific model or technique (Hubble et al., 1999). MI was developed to foster increased motivation based on respect and compassion within a relationship. Most importantly, motivation can be increased through this partnership and by conversations with a skilled MI practitioner (Thigpen et al., 2007). SDT does not explain all the variables for why people change, but it provides hints for when change is more likely to occur. (See Chapter 5 for a more in-depth review of SDT.)

Transtheoretical Model of Change

Both MI and coaching share an understanding of how people change. To address the question of how to help those "less ready to change," MI sought to determine the influences of motivation and how to combine those with the clinical style of MI. These factors are crucial when helping clients in the earlier stages of change.

Prochaska, Norcross, and DiClemente (1994) also sought to answer this question, and after combining important concepts from several models, they formulated the transtheoretical model of change (TTM). This model emerged in the 1980s, concurrent with the development of MI, and the two are compatible cousins. The TTM is a commonly used and well-researched model in behavioral change management (Hashemzadeh et al., 2019).

The TTM model describes five stages of change: precontemplation (no interest in making changes), contemplation (thinking about changing), preparation (preparing for change), action (recently taking steps to change), and maintenance (sustaining change over time). Knowing what methods and techniques are most effective for clients during each stage is vital, since you will want to adapt your approach based on their stage of change for that behavior. For example, if a client is stuck in contemplation about exercise, it would be unwise to prematurely create a goal to get to the gym 5 days a week. Readiness for a specific behavior is an essential factor, and if you fail to consider the client's readiness, your attempts to bypass the stage of change may poison further progress.

As we unwrap the strategies for effective coaching in later chapters, we will explain the stages of change in more detail. For now, it's important to recognize that most other methods are designed to help clients in the "I'm ready" stage of change. MI emerged partly to answer the question, "What about those clients who are less ready, who are in the 'I won't' or 'I can't' or 'I'm thinking about it' stage of change?" MI-informed coaching builds upon evidence-based methods to explore and empower clients to move through the stages of change.

Some people assume that MI is only applicable in the coaching process up until the point where clients have resolved their ambivalence or once they move beyond the contemplation stage. They argue that once a person is in the planning and action stage, MI is no longer needed. However, we believe this is a misunderstanding of the scope of MI. In future chapters, we will show how MI fits squarely onto the coaching model along the entire coaching process and sequence, from beginning to end.

EVIDENCE FOR EFFECTIVENESS OF MI

The vast number of studies around the topic of MI point to the ongoing interest in its application and potential effectiveness. Currently, there are over 2,000 controlled trials and studies and over 200 meta-analyses and systematic reviews on the effectiveness of MI. Many (but not all) investigations report positive outcomes using MI in the fields of addiction, education, health care, and behavioral health (Miller & Rollnick, 2023). An in-depth compilation of research for the evidence of the effectiveness of MI can be found online at *www.guilford.com/lanier-materials*.

Evidence for Effectiveness of Coaching with MI

If MI is shown to be effective, can we assume that coaching with MI produces equally positive results? The research is mounting to confirm that coaching with MI is effective. MI-informed coaching proved effective in diabetes care and disease management (Wan et al., 2018), helped increase quality of life, decreased depressive symptoms, and improved perceived stress scores (Clark et al., 2014). Coaching with MI was shown in one study to improve physical exercise habits, increase personal accountability and health awareness, and extend mindfulness practice for 2 years beyond the study (Benzo, 2013). Additionally, it helped to facilitate weight loss (Lancha et al., 2018), decrease body mass index, and encourage the client's readiness to change (Shahnazari et al., 2013). While MI is continually developing, new research and advances will likely continue to validate and improve MI's effectiveness and, thus, the effectiveness of coaching with MI.

As we reviewed these findings on coaching with MI, it became clear that incorporating MI into our coaching practice could be highly beneficial, especially since it aligns so well with the coach approach we defined in Chapter 1. We feel that this growing body of research begins to validate the methods, skills, and approach that MI-informed coaching brings to the profession of coaching. The lessons gleaned from these studies can help us develop and hone our coaching skills to benefit our clients and elevate the coaching profession overall. MI is continually developing, and new research will likely continue to validate and improve its effectiveness in coaching. Though MI has spread into various fields of service, we believe it aligns seamlessly with coaching and becomes not only an adjacent method but a foundational bedrock for the entire coaching paradigm.

Take It Further

Directions: Work with a partner or in your professional learning community to read and follow the instructions and respond to each of the questions below.

1. Locate Handout 2.1 online at *www.guilford.com/lanier-materials*. Read section 1, "A Sample Coach Checklist."
   a. Think back to one of your coaching sessions and answer the questions in the list.
   b. What questions might you add to help you gauge the success of your coaching session?
2. On Handout 2.1, read section 3, "Assessments." If you are familiar with either of the two assessments listed, please explain to others in your group how you might use these as informal assessments of client growth. (See Handout 5.3 for a blank Wheel of Life.)
3. On Handout 2.1, read sections 4 through 7. Choose one that appeals to you or one that you are curious about, and discuss with your group how you might use it to assess your client's growth.

Chapter 3

What Is Motivational Interviewing?

In Chapter 1, we explained the foundational concepts of the coach approach. We made the case that this way of helping people change is most effective when the coach first has the right heart and mindset. Coaching is something we do; the coach approach is the *way* we do it. MI, much like coaching, is both a method and a *way* of being and interacting with those who seek to change. As we enlarge upon MI's theory, methods, and strategies, we will show the direct parallels with coaching.

MI offers a shift in the approach to helping people change. This person-centered, collaborative, and goal-oriented way of communicating contrasts with a style that assumes the helper is the expert and the client needs direction and information with a solid prescribed path to follow. Instead, MI pays attention to the words spoken within the session, and the deeper beliefs and attitudes of the helper, while eliciting and strengthening the clients' language of change. Based on these beliefs, the MI practitioner calls forth the client's own motivation for change.

MI is a style designed to address the common issue of ambivalence about change. A focus develops as the helper elicits the person's own reasons for and commitment to specific goals. This process exists within a rich atmosphere of acceptance and compassion (Miller & Rollnick, 2023).

Notice how in the coach approach, we, too, describe coaching as a partnership seasoned by the coach's acceptance of, compassion for, and empowerment of the client. Like MI, coaching focuses on the client's exploration of their own motivation and commitment to set and accomplish goals for change. These goals relate to their own vision for improvement and those things that are most important in their life. As in MI, a coach supports a client in their ambivalence, normalizing this natural experience in the change process. These definitions of MI and the coach approach are entirely congruent. Much of the coaching strategies and the coach approach overall have emerged from the solid foundation provided by MI.

A BRIEF HISTORY OF MI

A discussion of the initiative and evolution of MI is incomplete without mention of the originator, Dr. William R. Miller. Miller's early training in both the client-centered counseling style of Carl Rogers and behavioral therapies combined with early research began to lay the path of discovery for MI (Miller & Rollnick, 2013).

Miller's work as a clinical psychologist focused on the treatment of addiction, an area fueled by his curiosity and exploration of the psychology of change. MI's infancy focused on the treatment of problem drinkers. What Miller saw in them seemed to contradict the prevailing and somewhat disparaging assumptions that the surrounding culture made about those who struggled with addiction. Miller did not find them to be pathological liars who lived in denial. Miller's instinct and personal beliefs drove him to test out an alternative, more humane, and respectful approach to helping those who struggled with alcohol.

Miller's early research (Miller et al., 1980) showed that empathic listening, also known as "accurate empathy," on the part of therapists resulted in the highest level of client success in managing their drinking. From this research, Miller and colleagues were able to predict the drinking outcomes of the clients for up to 2 years based simply on how well their counselor had listened. While all nine counselors in the study used the same manual-guided therapy, the outcomes for their clients were not the same. What made the difference? Those clients who worked with therapists who showed a high level of empathic skill had success in managing their drinking. This finding was repeated in an independent study a year later (Valle, 1981).

In fact, in a 2018 meta-analysis of 82 samples representing more than 6,000 clients, this one skill—a therapist's empathy—showed a strong correlation with client outcomes (Elliott et al., 2011; Elliott et al., 2018). Another study showed that therapists who demonstrate empathic skills are more likely to establish a partnership that predicts better outcomes (McClintock et al., 2019). The simple act of listening proved to be a powerful change agent.

That truth is foundational to coaching as well, and the coaching field has built upon this foundational research and premise. As we emphasized in Chapter 1, the coach approach is a prerequisite for more effective outcomes, and one key component of the coach approach is the skill of empathy.

Additionally, there are reverberating parallels in studies that show a strong association between a physician's level of empathy and patient outcomes. In one of many studies in the United States (Hojat et al., 2018), results showed that patients with diabetes whose physicians scored high on the empathy measurement scale were more likely to have good control of their A1c and LDL cholesterol compared to patients of physicians who scored low on the empathy scale. This shows the power of even a 15- to 20-minute office visit to impact patient improvement. Empathy, which includes listening well, is your starting point for helping people change and grow, in both MI and coaching.

The Evoking of MI

This impactful method, developed and further defined and explored by both Miller and Stephen Rollnick (2023), is currently in use across a diverse range of disciplines, such as career counseling, nursing, speech and language pathology, physical therapy, social work, sports psychology, executive coaching, school mental health counseling, career counseling, parole and probations, and correctional work, as well as life coaching, and health and wellness coaching. Despite its far-reaching influence today, MI began somewhat obscurely.

Shortly following his research findings on empathy, Miller moved to Norway and worked with a team of young psychologists to informally discuss treatment issues. He taught and demonstrated reflective listening skills while conducting role play with the psychologists, showing how the skills might be applied. The inquisitive learners had in-the-moment questions that emerged from their observations. These questions nudged Miller to verbalize and later define the principles or "decision rules" that seemed to guide his intuitive practice. The psychologists asked about the why, what, and how that influenced the methods. Over the weeks, Miller began to pen these principles, and shortly after that, they became the working definition of motivational interviewing (Miller, 1983).

The development of MI sprang forth from Miller's own intuitive practice and reflection. He credits the collaborative interaction between himself and those psychologists as the process that became the catalyst for the development of MI. He admits with a deliberate pun, "MI was literally evoked from me" (Miller & Rollnick, 2013, p. 373).

Discoveries in the Drinker's Checkup

Miller and associates designed a method called the Drinker's Checkup to increase the likelihood that drinkers would seek treatment after a single, brief intervention. The invitation was for drinkers to receive a free checkup to determine if alcohol was harmful to them. The surprising results showed that although few participants sought any help afterward, many participants significantly reduced their drinking even after the first brief session. Even more surprisingly, they maintained those gains in an 18-month follow-up. This simple approach seemed to motivate self-change in drinking, and clients appeared to make lasting changes in drinking even without follow-up interventions. The focus of MI then expanded from motivation for treatment to motivation for change.

Expanded studies of brief interventions for excessive drinking uncovered common factors for success. These factors included feedback, the responsibility of the client, offering options, using empathy, and providing support for self-confidence (Miller & Rollnick, 2013).

In this brief history of the origins of MI, there are consistent parallels to coaching. You use the coach approach by showing empathy, deeply listening while providing reflective feedback, exploring options, strengthening the client's self-confidence, and continually emphasizing your client's autonomy and responsibility.

THE SPIRIT OF MI: THE MISSING INGREDIENT

MI is a specific method with unique processes and components. It is a method whose skills can be taught and mastered, but as Miller and Rollnick began to train other practitioners in the use of MI, they saw an unwanted pattern developing. Something essential was missing. The therapies could sound hollow and dry, even though the therapists correctly used the skills.

The methods designed to engage and empower clients were instead feeling like something done *on* or *to* clients. The heart of the method was not beating as it should. But why? This curiosity led them to uncover and define the missing component, what they termed the "underlying spirit" of MI.

Undergirding the techniques is this spirit, the foundational heart and mindset that enrich the entire process, increasing its effectiveness. These components of partnership, acceptance, compassion, and empowerment help spark a connection from one human to another, a connection that enlivens and ignites client action. This spirit is something within a person and arises from assumptions and beliefs that drive thoughts, words, and actions. It is an essential perspective that gives voice and melody to the notes on the score. Without this spirit of MI, the unique potential of MI to help people may be severely limited or actually cause harm (Mohr, 1995; Moyers & Miller, 2013).

Imagine a chef who has all the ingredients for a recipe but fails to make a delicious dish. Just having the right ingredients is not enough. The chef must know how to create the perfect balance of flavors and textures. In the same way, we describe the coach approach as essential to effective coaching, and it sets the tone for every technique and tool you use. Without this coach approach, this spirit of MI, coaching might default to something akin to mentoring, teaching, advising, or just chatting among friends. While those have their place in the proper context, coaching's unique style, fashioned after MI, will not include those things very much, if at all.

At worst, failure to adopt this spirit of MI in coaching could render your session with a client little more than a dry intake of information to persuade or even manipulate the client into making a change. We know that does not work. The spirit of MI makes the techniques effective, and this spirit is a vital prerequisite for helping people change.

You, as a coach, can be relieved to know that you do not have to wait until you master this spirit before beginning MI practice. This spirit is something that can be developed and honed through intentional focus.

THE SPIRIT OF MI AND THE COACH APPROACH

As we mentioned above, the spirit of MI includes the four elements of partnership, acceptance, compassion, and empowerment. In our early training as coaches, we were surprised to learn how closely MI and coaching were aligned. The criteria standards for coaching, defined by the content outline in the NBHWC and the core competencies of the ICF, correlate directly or indirectly to the methods, skills, and approach of MI.

We will make more explicit connections between MI and coaching, and we will refer to the NBHWC and the ICF within the discussion of each component of MI. As we discussed in Chapter 1, these organizations set the criteria standards and the core competencies that define and standardize coaching practice. You will see how the MI components, including the tasks, skills, and specific methods, apply to coaching. More elaboration will be forthcoming in later chapters.

BOX 3.1. The Coaches' CAPE

Compassion: intentionally putting your clients' needs first, embracing the worth of each individual, and taking action to promote your clients' needs.

Acceptance: seeing and accepting each client as they are, withholding judgment, and acting on the belief that your clients are creative, resourceful, and whole.

Partnership: forming a trusting relationship where you work together to co-create goals and solutions that are important to your client.

Empowerment: acknowledging and eliciting your clients' motivations, desires, abilities, reasons, and needs for change.

For the coach, we have taken the liberty to arrange the four components of the spirit of MI to form the acronym CAPE. This may remind you to don the coaches' CAPE—the spirit of MI—each time you interact with your clients. (See Box 3.1, The Coaches' CAPE.)

MI Spirit: Compassion

Miller and Rollnick (2023) described compassion as something other than a sympathetic feeling, as more than suffering with the troubles of clients. Compassion is an intention to give deference to and actively promote the clients' needs.

Compassion is foundational to all the other therapeutic skills. So, too, in coaching, you are careful to demonstrate compassion by building genuine respect and rapport with your clients. These are musts for effective coach–client relationships. See the coach sample below for how you might use the spirit of compassion in the coaching relationship.

Coaching Sample: What Might Compassion Look Like in Coaching?

A client worked with a coach after a major health scare and a referral from his physician. He wanted to make lifestyle changes to help him recover from complications such as kidney disease and prediabetes. At the end of a 12-week coaching relationship, he reached his goals of walking daily, eating healthy foods, keeping a gratitude journal, and reducing stress by reframing negative thinking. He was even able to stop taking a few medications because of his excellent progress.

But several weeks after the sessions ended, the client was surrounded by a former crowd of friends, and he fell back into old, harmful habits. He had a recurrence of symptoms, was admitted to the hospital, and was headed for a significant relapse. The coach, first unaware of the situation, messaged her client for a routine 4-week follow-up. Once the coach realized the gravity of the problem, she felt disappointed and even judgmental toward her client. Instead of responding immediately, she spent a few days reframing her thinking.

The coach challenged herself, "Why do I feel judgmental?" and "Why do I want to express disappointment about how he got in this predicament?" She remembered the C in CAPE (compassion), and instead of the negative judgments, she posed a new set of questions.

"How can I promote his well-being?"
"How can I show compassion by helping him in this challenge?"
"How can I act to help alleviate his suffering?"

The shift toward compassion sparked a new perspective and a desire to act. The coach remembered the spirit of compassion and began considering ways to support instead of judge her client. What do you suppose would have been the result if the coach had maintained a negative, judgmental, and disappointed stance? Below is the resulting conversation between the coach and client in messages over the next few days.

COACH: I heard you're back home from the hospital and having some challenges. I wonder if you'd be interested in starting our coaching sessions again. [*Careful to avoid judgment in any way.*]

CLIENT: I'm doing fine, and I am back on track. I'll let you know if I need coaching. I can't afford to buy healthy food right now because I need to get back on the medications. [*Client ambivalence and hesitancy.*]

COACH: [Several days later.] Hello again! The invitation is open to come just as you are if you'd like to restart coaching at any time. [*No conditions for "getting things right" before coming to coaching.*]

CLIENT: [*Five minutes later.*] How about Monday? [*The client felt safe and welcome to come back even after temporarily lapsing.*]

Coach's Reflection

The coach knew the client was not "fine" but felt it was important to honor his autonomy. She understood that her response could foster or hinder her client's motivation to reengage efforts for change. How did the coach offer help? She gave him space, showed respect and positive regard, and acknowledged his personal choice to do what he thought was best. The coach made the offer for coaching sessions without judgment. The client's quick response to the invitation was—the coach believes—a result of demonstrating compassion.

MI Spirit: Acceptance

The lovely child is easier to love, and the compliant client is a pleasure. But the attitude of acceptance implies that sometimes people come with unpleasant qualities, reluctance, or tangled and complex circumstances. Just how important is it to feel and express acceptance for your clients? All clients?

Carl Rogers held that acceptance is fundamental to healing. He recognized that feeling unaccepted might be the impetus for people to become immobilized and remain unchanged (Rogers, 1951). Acceptance includes a complete acceptance of what the client brings, which differs from approval.

Acceptance is more than being tolerant. It is fully seeing what is there while simultaneously and intentionally withholding judgment. When you witness someone languishing in what appear to be harmful habits or repeated failed attempts, your passion for helping them could stir up evaluative judgments.

If so, it may be helpful to remember that the person in front of you is most likely aware of their stubborn habits or diminished life. They may have been made to feel bad, guilty, or shamed into changing. As contrary as it seems, those judgments from others have most likely failed to produce any real and lasting change. In MI and coaching, you understand the power of accepting people precisely as they are, unconditionally. It is often within the context of this paradox that the changer finds the courage and motivation to change.

Your Beliefs Are Showing: Theory X and Y

What a person believes about other people has consequences. Leadership theory identified Theories X and Y to describe contrasting views of human nature. This work by Douglas McGregor (2006) applied to management, but we can see the implications in the helping professions more generally. Theory X conveys the belief that people are inherently lazy and need to be coerced or threatened to get something done. People lack self-regulation and therefore need rewards and penalties in place. Conversely, Theory Y conveys the belief that people are capable of self-direction, have creativity and resourcefulness, and will flourish when given the right environment. Both Theory X and Theory Y managers adjust their styles based on what they believe about the workers, and both find that their beliefs come true.

How do you, as a coach, demonstrate a fundamental element of acceptance? How do you show your truest acceptance of clients in an authentic and believable way? You, too, like managers, will likely treat clients as your beliefs dictate.

The acceptance component of the spirit of MI is further defined by four subtopics: absolute worth, autonomy support, accurate empathy, and affirmation.

MI Spirit: Acceptance—Absolute Worth

MI defines "absolute worth" as a nonjudgmental attitude that values persons as they are and refuses to impose conditions on their worth (Rogers, 1980).

In Chapter 1, we repeated the firmly held coach belief: Our clients are creative, resourceful, and whole. This belief is not just a feeling; it is a foundational assumption, and your successful coaching practice is built upon this repertoire of thoughts, words, and actions. You must believe clients are whole, not broken. They have the potential to grow and actualize to become their best selves. Once people feel accepted in this way, it frees them to change.

MI Spirit: Acceptance—Accurate Empathy

The descriptor "accurate" implies that sometimes your attempts to show empathy are less than on target. If you see a person in distress, and your first response is to tell them a story about your suffering, you might miss the mark. Likewise, if you put your arm around a client's shoulders and confirm that you know how they feel, you may be making a risky guess about their internal perspective. One can see the many ways your arrows may shoot way beyond or too short of the bullseye. Fully understanding your clients is a way of showing your acceptance of them.

In MI, accurate empathy is about understanding the other's perspective and seeing the world through their eyes. To understand people's inner world, it is wise to withhold assumptions and instead actively seek to understand their experiences or feelings.

Accurate empathy is a skill that can be learned, and we will explicitly show how to use those MI techniques in coaching in later chapters. Initially, it may be worthwhile to examine your assumptions about your clients' internal views.

As coaches, you listen deeply to understand, expand, and then offer reflections to demonstrate your understanding of clients' perspectives. During focused conversation, clients often discover what is deep inside.

MI Spirit: Acceptance—Autonomy Support

A key concept in MI is that since clients are free to choose what to do with their lives, helpers are most effective when they acknowledge and support this autonomy. When helpers try to make people do or want to do something, the result is usually reluctance and holding to the status quo. MI reminds helpers to let go of that perceived power over another individual (Miller & Rollnick, 2013).

One of the primary desired effects of MI is for clients to drop a defensive stance. When clients are reluctant, one can predict the probable outcome; they cling to the status quo. Paradoxically, change can begin when a person's autonomy and freedom of choice are acknowledged.

Coaching builds upon the same assumption about autonomy. Admittedly, it can be a surprising discovery for new coaches to find that they will need to lay aside their expert hat and allow the client to exercise autonomy. But soon, the power of this approach is revealed when you begin to glimpse the light of the client's own inner genius shining through.

MI Spirit: Acceptance—Affirmation

Affirmation in MI is an intentional way of finding and acknowledging the client's strengths and efforts, both something the person has done as well as enduring attributes. This way of demonstrating acceptance shifts the focus from seeing what is wrong with people to highlighting what is right and good.

In coaching, affirmation includes using positive psychology. Like in MI, you focus on your clients' character strengths, acknowledge their efforts, encourage experimentation and learning versus trial and error, and help them reframe negative thinking patterns. You are prizing the clients regardless of their behavior, in keeping with acceptance. You are giving approval and respect as a fundamental human right, not withholding it until they earn it.

MI Spirit: Partnership

MI asserts that a collaborative relationship between helper and client is more effective than a directive, expert-led approach. After all, counseling and psychotherapy deal with behavior and lifestyle, not broken bones or reconstructive surgery. In those instances, the surgeon hardly needs the patient's opinion and expertise in anatomy and surgical technique. Unlike the surgeon and patient, the helper in a counseling or coaching relationship relies on the active engagement of the client. No one is more well-versed in the client's narrative and reasons for change than the client. No one knows their unique motivational factors like the client does, and no one is an expert on the client except the client. To foster people's change, you need to call upon their expertise and engagement. This partnership helps to ensure engagement.

It can be a bit of a jolt to discover that you will take off the expert hat as a coach. But within the context of honoring your client's expertise and autonomy, you will likely find your comfort zone. You will still bring information, ideas, and your unique expertise in coaching and other fields to the coaching session. But this offering is done in a particular way. When given permission, or when clients ask you for information, you will offer your expertise in the correct dose, at the right moment, for the benefit of the client. In this partnership, both you and the client are experts.

By taking off your expert hat, you mirror the MI belief that partnership is the construct that works best because human beings make their own choices about how to live and flourish. You echo the truth that any efforts to force change in others can have a negative countereffect (Brehm & Brehm, 2013; de Almeida Neto, 2017; Karno & Longabaugh, 2005).

MI Spirit: Empowerment

The hallmark of MI echoes resoundingly in this element of empowerment. It is here that MI's song rings its powerful message. Beneath this melody is the counterculture belief that spurred the unique approach more than three decades ago. The humble beginnings of this method invite you to continue in humility and curiosity as you seek to support people's change and growth. It is here where Miller's original conundrum finds its resolve. When society declared that those who struggled with alcohol were inherently irresponsible and liars, Miller created a new narrative driven by respect and hope.

As a coach, you also understand that people already have what is needed to change and grow to their potential. Empowerment acknowledges a client's choice and ability, as well as their own reasons for change. It is your humble privilege to unlock your client's power to begin the path of discovery toward their own wisdom and ability. You empower them with the gift of your genuine curiosity, hope, and expectation that they can and will uncover and release their unique inner genius.

The spirit of MI and the coach approach are not strategies coaches can pull out and memorize. They are not steps to take along a continuum of mastery. They are attitudes of heart and mind that coaches can continually foster with intentional awareness and practice. As we later unfold the how-to of coaching with MI and explore the methods, skills, and strategies, we encourage you to embrace and demonstrate these necessary attitudes constantly; put on your CAPE. The spirit of MI is the thread woven throughout the entire tapestry of coaching. The more you notice and raise your awareness of these heart and mindset attitudes, the more you will find ways to incorporate them into every session with your clients. Many coaches admit that this way of thinking and interacting with people has influenced more than their work with clients. It is a profoundly powerful way to live.

SHARED ASSUMPTIONS ABOUT CHANGE

The Helpers' Mindset

MI and coaching share assumptions about change and the changer. First, the MI spirit and the coach approach (CAPE) describe a way of *being* with clients and, as we stated earlier, a mindset shift that is growth-oriented versus fixed in a pattern of ideas.

This MI spirit—the coaching mindset—invites you to approach your coaching clients with curiosity and humility. Instead of having a hidden agenda for them, you understand that they are the experts in their own lives, and with your guidance, they can find the solutions that are best for them. This, in turn, influences the types of conversations you have with your clients.

The MI coach serves as an ally and works in a respectful partnership with clients. You view clients as worthy of respect, as people who embody both strengths and weaknesses, who have personal values, hopes, and a developing sense of vision. You bring your own expertise to the table while also emphasizing and drawing forth your clients' expertise, creativity, and potential, not their brokenness and failure.

The ICF core competencies (2019) succinctly summarize the coaching mindset as "open, curious, flexible, and client-centered." The eight subcompetencies of ICF core competency 1 (demonstrates ethical practice) point to coaches' need for ongoing personal and professional growth to enhance their skills, stressing that coaches should develop reflective practice. You strive to be increasingly aware of your own intuition, your ability to regulate your emotions, and the influences of culture on yourself and others. With humility, you, as a coach, will seek help from outside sources when you feel it benefits your clients. (See Table 3.1 on pp. 46–47 for a summary of the CAPE mindset shifts.)

The Guiding Style

Another shared assumption about change is the style of conversations used in sessions. MI conversations follow a guiding style that is illustrated as a midway point on a continuum between leading and following. *Leading* is at one extreme where the helper assumes the responsibility of dispensing knowledge and direction to the client. The result could be that the client becomes somewhat passive and unengaged. *Following* is at the other end of the continuum, where the helper becomes minimally involved, trusting clients to work things out on their own. (See Figure 3.1.)

Coaching also uses the guiding style, though both leading and following styles are used with clients at various times throughout many helper relationships, including coaching. For example, clients who may have exhausted their resources in finding solutions may need and ask for your direction. Conversely, clients who are more ready to change and are already reaching many goals may require less and less of your input when reflecting on and designing new goals.

In between the two extremes, guiding is where MI conversations and coaching usually land. This is where you and your clients work together in a partnership to share ideas, brainstorm, consider options, co-create, and reflect on progress and learning.

Guiding does not imply that you simply observe or nod with polite agreement. Neither are you leading the charge by overly suggesting, teaching, informing, or persuading clients. You guide them to get where they want to go and collaborate on the best path to arrive at the destination. You focus on the growth and development of your clients with a view toward their autonomy and self-regulation.

A helpful analogy for a guiding style can be found in the teaching–learning model of instruction. Initially, teachers are more involved and spend high-level efforts demonstrating, explaining, clarifying, and talking to the learners. The learners, in contrast, are receivers who observe, listen, and are—at first—less verbal and involved than their teachers. Teachers do most of the work in this shorter "leading" phase.

TABLE 3.1. CAPE Mindset Shifts (Coach Approach)

From this mindset →	To this mindset
Sympathy	*Compassion*
• Sympathizing and showing pity for your clients' dilemmas.	• Seeking to explore and understand your clients' perspectives.
• Rescuing your clients and encouraging their compliance.	• Trusting in your clients' capabilities and inspiring self-discovery and learning.
• Persuading your clients that you have what they need to improve.	• Actively seeking your clients' best interest, regardless of your approval.
• Sharing your own experiences to help clients see your perspective.	• Listening to understand more of your clients' narratives, not your narratives.
Judgment	*Acceptance*
• Assigning value to your clients and their actions.	• Accepting your clients' value, regardless of their actions.
• Feeling and expressing approval or disapproval of your clients' actions.	• Respecting your clients just as they are, without conditions for acceptance.
• Establishing conditions for clients to be successful and worthy of your approval.	• Demonstrating unconditional regard for clients regardless of their attempts.
• Making assumptions about your clients' situations.	• Showing empathy by seeking to understand your clients' dilemmas.
• Working hard to get your clients to work on goals you choose.	• Encouraging clients to work on goals they choose, that are important to them.
• Praising clients for their compliance.	• Identifying and affirming your clients' strengths and efforts.
• Seeing and trying to fix what is wrong with your clients.	• Seeing clients as whole and capable of solving their own problems.
• Setting the agenda for your clients.	• Accepting clients' choices and agendas.
Leadership	*Partnership*
• Believing that clients need your expertise to make changes.	• Believing in and supporting your clients' expertise in themselves.
• Taking charge and telling your clients what to focus on for change.	• Collaborating on options for change while emphasizing clients' autonomy.
• Persuading clients to choose the "right" way to change.	• Working alongside clients to explore choices for what and how to change.
• Telling clients what is necessary for their progress.	• Encouraging clients to take a journey of self-discovery and learning.
• Setting rewards and consequences for motivating your clients.	• Engaging with clients to uncover their own motivations and reasons for change.

(continued)

TABLE 3.1. *(continued)*

From this mindset →	To this mindset
Instruction	***Empowerment***
• Giving your clients a clear plan to help them get "unstuck."	• Drawing out the resources and ideas that are within your clients.
• Determining your clients' deficit to be corrected.	• Identifying your clients' strengths to be leveraged.
• Motivating your clients by showing the pros and cons of changing.	• Evoking your clients' own reasons and motivations for changing.
• Explaining to your clients how they landed in their current dilemmas.	• Seeking to understanding your clients' perspective about their dilemmas.
• Noticing and deciding which problems prevent your clients from changing.	• Noticing and affirming your clients' strengths, past efforts, unique qualities.
• Planning your clients' path to compliance toward change.	• Supporting your clients' self-regulation toward lasting change.

Next comes the "guiding" phase, where learners gradually try out things for themselves. They experiment, verbalize, problem-solve, and grapple with new ideas; they are more actively engaged. The teacher's role evolves as an equally engaged partner, walking alongside learners to guide, clarify, reflect, and point the work and the learner toward the learning targets. While allowing for increased independence on the part of learners, teachers remain close by to support, encourage, or redirect as needed, often in the form of verbal feedback.

The end goal, the "following" phase, is for learners to eventually demonstrate independence by applying the new learning and skills within novel contexts. In this final phase, teachers take a more diminished presence and become less directive while they foster the learners' burgeoning new understanding. Learners are the most actively engaged in this phase, while the less engaged teachers observe and follow.

To follow this analogy, in MI-consistent sessions, coaches primarily work in the "guiding" style of partnership and shared engagement with the client. Of course, there will be times during your coaching relationship when you may lean more toward following, such as the initial part of engaging. (Engaging is the topic of Chapter 4). During that time, you establish your relationship, develop trust and rapport, and let your clients experience what it is like to have their coach listen to them deeply and without judgment. Likewise, there are times when it may be appropriate to use a more directive, "leading" style, such as when clients want more specific information or ask where to find resources for fleshing out a doctor's prescription to "manage stress."

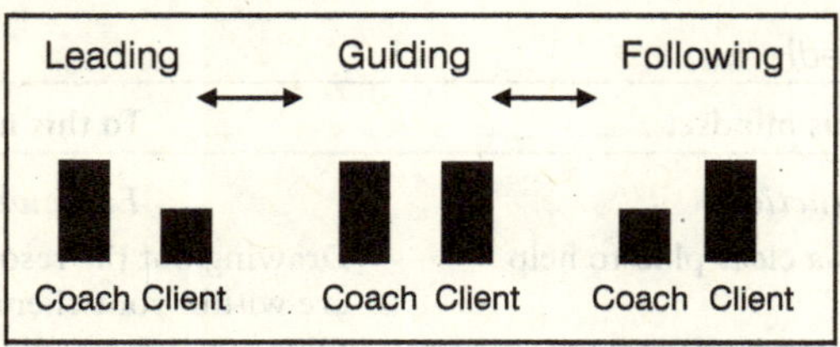

FIGURE 3.1. A continuum of helper styles. The bars indicate the coach's and client's relative engagement in the process.

However, most of the time, you will be guiding clients along their journey of growth and discovery. We will talk more about this in upcoming chapters when we describe the methods in more detail. Figure 3.1 shows the relative level of engagement of the coach and the client in the leading, guiding, and following styles.

MOTIVATION

MI and coaching share assumptions about motivation, a pivotal concept in MI. Later, we unwrap the how-to of coaching with MI and explore ways to stir up and draw forth clients' motivations to change. But here, we draw attention to a few shared premises about motivation that are driving forces for the techniques used in MI.

Ambivalence

Everyone is motivated by something, whether to keep a habit or behavior or to remove that habit or behavior. This wanting of two opposing realities is described as ambivalence and is often experienced as an uncomfortable volley of internal self-talk. You can hear the types of language expressed by the client, described as sustain talk and change talk. You may hear clients argue for staying the same (sustain talk) or give reasons for changing the behavior (change talk) within the same conversation. The MI style of communication is designed to draw forth these arguments so clients can hear their own reasons for change and resolve their ambivalence.

The motivation to stay comfortable in the status quo (sustain) is often the stronger side of the pros-and-cons debate in a person's internal struggle. But once these arguments come to light, either side—sustain talk or change talk—can exert a powerful force on the person's commitment to change. Hearing oneself verbalize the reasons to change is a significant impetus for moving forward; people are empowered by what they hear themselves say.

Although ambivalence is not a pathology but a normal part of change, you will want to use caution to avoid focusing too much attention on your clients' sustain talk and their arguments for staying the same. Studies indicate that the amount of change talk compared to sustain talk influences the subsequent change. If your clients voice more change talk than sustain talk, they are more likely to change, and the opposite is also true (Glynn & Moyers, 2010).

The language clients offer on the side of change during MI sessions is considered a key component for change. MI research asserts that clients decide about their unwanted behavior as they verbalize their thoughts and therefore talk themselves into change (Moyers et al., 2009). Based on this assertion, MI designed the MI method for evoking clients' talk in favor of change rather than talk of staying the same.

The success of this process relies on the clients' genuine and spontaneous expression of their reasons for making a change. Their spontaneity depends on the trusting relationship you build and the safe and judgment-free zone you provide. The power of their own words convinces them about their behavior and is a vital ingredient in MI practice. The conversation is gently guided so that clients offer reasons for change and come face-to-face with their ambivalence (Moyers et al., 2009). (This skill is further explored in Chapter 6.)

As we have already mentioned, the ambivalent person is often stuck between two opposing forces. This discomfort may be why coaching clients hesitate, remain stuck, or convince themselves that the situation is not that bad or that they have run out of options, especially if they have already tried and failed.

Emotions such as fear of failure or uncertainty about one's ability to succeed are possible factors that keep people from moving past the status quo. If you hope your ambivalent client will be vulnerable and feel free to share and explore their reasons for change, you will remember your CAPE. You will create an environment of compassion and acceptance where you listen with a nonjudgmental ear.

Internal versus External Motivation

When people try to change, they often say they do not have enough motivation. The problem may not be the amount of motivation but the *type* of motivation that is lacking.

Sometimes people have external pressures to change. "If you don't quit smoking, your lung disease and cancer risk raise significantly, and your COPD will only worsen." For some, this will spark the needed change, but for others, it may take more than that, or rather, it may take a different kind of motivation.

People need to connect to their internal drivers for change and their intrinsic motivations. When people connect their goals to their personal values, purpose, and meaning, this can stir their intrinsic motivation. The good news is that intrinsic motivation is associated with longer-lasting changes (DiClemente et al., 1999).

Both internal and external forces influence motivation. Some clients seek help from coaches because of a mandate from an employer or doctor, and this pressure gets the momentum going for them. "I want to learn to control my temper so that I can keep my job" or "I have to lose weight so I can have this knee surgery." These clients choose to avoid negative consequences, but this short-range view is often a detour from long-term changes. Although behavior changes can occur for external reasons, the change is often short-lived (Ryan & Deci, 2000). To help clients make lasting changes, MI uses techniques that access clients' internal motivations.

Take It Further

Directions: Discuss items 1–3 with your learning community. Then, work together to answer item 4. Finally, work independently to write your answer to item 5.

1. The coaches' CAPE (spirit of MI) is the *way* you do everything else you do. Name the four components of CAPE and explain how adopting this heart and mindset can affect your coaching practice.
2. Locate and read items 1–3 on "Shared Assumptions about Change" (Handout 3.1 at *www.guilford.com/lanier-materials*). Discuss some practical ways that these assumptions can positively impact your coaching.
3. Refer to item 4 on Handout 3.1. Discuss how you might use an MI-consistent coach approach with clients in each of the five stages of change. (See Chapter 5 for more on the stages of change.)
4. Locate the ICF Professional Certified Coach Credentials and Standards (You'll find a link to those credentials and standards at *www.guilford.com/lanier-materials*.) Make a list of each competency and corresponding marker that relates to MI, either directly or indirectly. Do the same for the NBHWC Practical Skills Guidelines. (You'll find a link to those guidelines at *www.guilford.com/lanier-materials*.)
5. Read and reflect on the following statement, then expand on it and write it in your own words. *The MI spirit, principles, and methods lay the foundation for our coaching practice; it is a golden thread woven throughout coaching.*

Part II

Practicing Motivational Interviewing in Coaching

This book is about coaching with MI. We explored the foundational beliefs and theories of MI and coaching in Part I. In Part II, we explicitly connect the MI methods, tasks, and skills to coaching by emphasizing the convergence between the two. We often refer to the relevant standards for coaching practice from the NBHWC (2020) and the core competencies from the ICF (2019b) alongside the discussion of MI tasks and skills.

THE FOUR TASKS AND FOUR CORE SKILLS OF MI

The four MI tasks, defined as engaging, focusing, evoking, and planning, describe a general order of things that facilitates the process of helping people change and grow. While these are naturally sequential, they are not meant to be rigid. You will find yourselves moving in and out of the four tasks. However, each task includes a unique application of the MI methods and skills that help structure the conversation in a particular way for a specific purpose. These four MI tasks also become the foundation for coaching practice.

Engaging

Engagement is a prerequisite for establishing the necessary connection between the client and the helper in the initial stages, and it remains vital throughout all four tasks. Taking the time to develop a good connection is worth the investment, and without it, the subsequent processes are unlikely to be effective. The relationship is foundational to MI-consistent coaching.

Focusing

Focusing comes next with a more directional (not directive) intent, moving the conversation toward the client's agenda. MI coaches remember that engagement, or establishing trust and rapport, as coaches say, is a means to an end. You are going somewhere in the focusing process, and clients are more likely to reach the destination if you have worked with the client to pin a flag to the map. Clients have come to get help moving forward.

Evoking

Evoking is the task that sets MI apart from other methods; it is the heart of MI and coaching. The MI practitioner or coach skillfully elicits the clients' own ideas about why and how to change once you two have chosen a focus. The purpose is to have clients voice their own arguments for change and to empower your clients to reflect on, verbalize, and uncover their own motivations for change.

Planning

Planning occurs when there seems to be sufficient motivation to move forward, and the conversation shifts to working out the particulars of when and how the change will happen. As you work together, you pay close attention to eliciting the clients' own solutions while respecting their autonomy.

Figure PII depicts the four tasks of MI in graphic form. We added opening and closing bookends, which we will elaborate on in Chapter 14. For now, notice how the engaging task continues as a foundation for the entire process of the conversation.

FOUR CORE SKILLS

Coaching with MI requires a set of attitudes and then a collection of skills through which the attitudes are materialized. As we said, core skills are employed throughout all four tasks of MI and in coaching. These are foundational skills to be developed as one seeks to be proficient. The first four

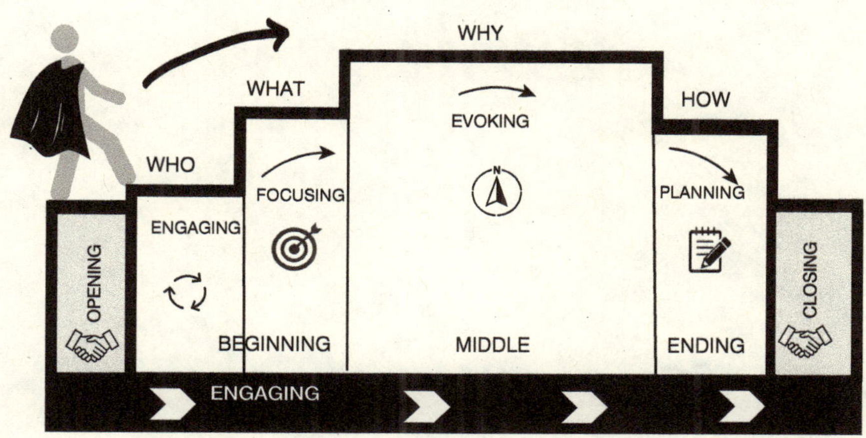

FIGURE PII. The four tasks of MI.

skills form the acronym OARS: open questions, affirmations, reflections, and summaries. (Chapter 4 addresses the four skills.) An additional skill is informing and advising, which may seem contradictory in a client-centered approach at first glance. However, sharing information is appropriate when the client asks for it or when the helper has asked permission to share. Still, it is essential to continue honoring clients' autonomy as you offer the information and to remember clients are experts in themselves. This topic is covered in more detail in Chapter 8.

These skills find their roots in other person-centered approaches (Hill, 2009; Ivey et al., 2009). What is unique to MI is that these skills are used within the context of the spirit of MI to evoke and empower the client to choose and design change. The same can be said for the coach approach. These skills are not tips and tricks used to manipulate people; these are effective, well-researched, and proven best practices that prioritize engagement for the client's benefit.

Chapter 4

The Engaging Task and Four Core Motivational Interviewing Skills

Although influenced by the Rogerian client-centered approach, MI is somewhat more directional than what is typically thought of as a Rogerian style. This directionality is achieved through a guiding style of conversation and is also used in the goal-oriented coaching style.

THE GUIDING STYLE

As we discussed in Chapter 3, MI uses the guiding style throughout all tasks of MI as the most effective way to facilitate change and growth. Coaches are guides also as they walk alongside clients in the journey toward change. This guiding style is focused on engaging clients to become increasingly active and participatory in the coaching partnership. Directing, guiding, and following are all used by helpers and practitioners to some extent. However, the middle ground between directing and following is the guiding style, and this middle ground is primarily where MI and coaching exist. MI practitioners and coaches are client-centered but more directional than the following style and less expert-driven than the directing style (Miller & Rollnick, 2023). Guiding clients involves empowering them to choose their own paths while pointing them in the right directions.

As the introduction to Part II states, throughout this book we will refer to some of the relevant standards from the NBHWC and the core competencies from the ICF. In discussing the engaging task, these standards are germane. The NBHWC emphasizes a client-centered relationship where the coach acts a facilitator to empower clients to self-discover the personal values, resources, and strategies that are meaningful. ICF competency D.8 points to facilitating client growth as a coach "partners with the client to transform learning insight into action" and "promotes client autonomy in the coaching process." This facilitation can be achieved in a guiding (not leading) style.

THE ENGAGING TASK

The success of the guiding style is entirely dependent upon the relationship built between helper and client. Engaging is the first task, but it also depicts what happens within this task and is the natural prerequisite for everything that follows in the relationship. This alliance between the helper and the client determines the success of client outcomes (Flückiger et al., 2020). A respectful, collaborative, and ethically sound approach makes a difference. Within the first few minutes clients can decide whether a coach provides a safe environment and will genuinely hear them and try to understand their perspective.

Skimming over the act of engagement may cause later techniques to feel disconnected, like metal bolts rattling in an empty tin can. The most essential task in both MI and coaching is building a relationship of genuine connection with your client. Once that is established, techniques used within the context of this engagement become powerful tools to help guide clients toward their desired goals.

Engagement begins with the initial exchange between you and the client. Clients seeking help want to know if they will be listened to and respected and if you will understand their perspectives. They will want assurance that the alliance is one of mutual trust and respect. Engagement is vital to maintain throughout all tasks, and although it may become weakened at times, it is possible to restrengthen it at any point.

What you do is important, but how you do it is most important. Successful client outcomes directly relate to the value of the working relationship—clients' engagement—with the helper (Crits-Christoph et al., 2011). You can become better at engaging by improving listening skills, recognizing strengths, and emphasizing autonomy. This conveys to clients your belief that they are whole, not broken, and that you see them as people with inherent worth, strengths, and a capacity for change. In coaching terminology, this engagement task is defined as developing trust and rapport.

The NBHWC standards emphasize trust and rapport that are built in a positive and safe environment where your clients feel accepted and supported. Within this safety, clients can be honest and vulnerable and better access the values and motivations they need. Furthermore, your confidence in the clients' abilities to learn, grow, and change supports your clients' self-efficacy.

The ICF competencies also echo the importance of the coach–client relationship, which we propose is achieved through a guiding approach.

> ICF B.4.1–6—Cultivates trust and safety. "Partners with the client to create a safe, supportive environment that allows the client to share freely. Maintains a relationship of mutual respect and trust."

The best way to engage (or reengage) with clients is to do so with empathic listening and reflections to uncover the clients' meaning behind their words. This engagement is essential as both an initial and an ongoing component within a positive coach–client relationship. It is perpetuated by a deep respect for clients and continuous careful listening that honors their preferences and needs.

> ICF C.6.1–6—Listens actively. "Focuses on what the client is and is not saying to fully understand what is being communicated in the context of the client systems and to support client self-expression."

THE ROLE OF EMPATHY IN THE ENGAGING TASK

As mentioned at the beginning of this chapter, the focus on empathic listening originates from Carl Rogers's client-centered approach (Rogers, 1951). Empathy is the ability to perceive your clients' views and feelings, sharpen your understanding of their perspectives, and relate that understanding back to them through reflections. Much emphasis is on using empathic listening to do MI well, since research shows that empathy is a decisive predictor of outcomes across a variety of behaviors (McClintock et al., 2019).

Are people born with empathy? Do some of us possess a greater capacity for empathy? Maybe so, but if not, there are ways to build and practice one's capacity for it, wherever you may land on the spectrum of being empathic. Learning reflective listening can help you strengthen empathy.

Thomas Gordon (1970) described this skill as "active listening," which is entirely different than sitting back with quiet agreement. It is not sympathy either, which tends to focus on sharing a person's own experience. It may include acknowledging emotions while maintaining a separate perspective. Active listening is an intentional practice of listening to your clients and then offering reflective statements to build trust and connection.

The NBHWC competencies further clarify trust and rapport as paying attention to the clients' emotions as well as their words and behaviors. To practice active listening, you will use curiosity, mindful presence, and nonjudgment to become aware of what is happening with your client and yourself. Self-management will help you refrain from "knowing" what your client needs. Instead, these competencies emphasize allowing clients time and space to reflect, process, and make discoveries. Being attentive, open-minded, and curious without making assumptions will allow you to demonstrate empathy by pacing your communication to fit your clients' needs and listening for what is not being said.

The NBHWC competencies stress that active listening is more than allowing silence. A coach conveys "I'm hearing you" by offering reflections. These statements allow clients to see their own words, perspectives, and beliefs. Use of nonjudgmental reflections engages clients and inspires learning. Similarly, ICF competency B.5.1 points to the practice of active listening: "Remains focused, observant, empathetic, and responsive to the client."

Empathy in the Engaging Task

Here is an example of what empathy looks like in a coaching session.

CLIENT: I would like to have more clarity on how I'm approaching my new business. It needs to be aligned with who I am. I don't know if I have enough of myself to do all I need to do.

COACH: You want clarity, bottom line. Why is clarity important to you?

CLIENT: The reason I'm creating my business is to create work that's aligned with my values. If I'm not clear, then I lack direction. I feel like I'm being pulled in too many directions. I need to make decisions while taking it all into consideration.

COACH: It's a time to make big decisions. You want to make sure you're considering everything, especially since you recently left a job where you weren't happy. You want your new business to align with who you are as a person. What do you think we need to look at today?

The coach uses empathic listening by respectfully listening and emphasizing the client's autonomy. The coach offers simple reflections and a short summary to demonstrate that they are listening to the client. The coach also allows the client to choose the topic of the session. The open-ended questions will enable the client to reflect further and explore their values and motivations for making this change.

EARLY TRAPS IN ENGAGING

Forming an equal partnership seems straightforward. Although the coach can accomplish this early and quickly, some approaches could tilt the balance of power and put the client in a more passive role. The goal for

MI-consistent coaches is to engage an active client in the partnership and thereby increase the likelihood of change. A significant impediment to engaging is the implication that the coach is in the driver's seat. Miller and Rollnick (2013) identify six possible traps that threaten to take the client out of an active role and stifle the engagement.

The Assessment Trap

Relying too much on intake assessments may prove counterproductive to the engaging task. A series of written assessments could jeopardize the client's active involvement and instead invite passivity. It could send the message that the one who asks the questions is superior to the one who answers. Instead of leading the session with fact-gathering assessment reviews, allow clients to voice their own narratives and explore their dilemmas in the audience of a caring and skillful listener. The positive result is the unfolding of more profound and nuanced stories and information about the client that might have been overlooked on an assessment form. In this space, the clients are allowed to explore their deeper values and overall vision for their lives.

The NBHWC-related competencies parallel this approach by stating that coaches should spend time in the early session(s) exploring a client's values, vision, and purpose. By spending enough time exploring your client's understanding of their health and wellness goals, you prevent setting goals prematurely.

ICF competency C.6.1 also describes a coach's effort to understand the client: "Considers the client's context, identity, environment, experiences, values, and beliefs to enhance understanding of what the client is communicating."

The Expert Trap

Removing the expert hat frees you to approach and communicate with clients within the context of a partnership. You allow clients to discover and express their own expertise. Otherwise, it may be tempting to assume that once enough of the right information is collected, you can offer expert solutions to your clients. In MI-consistent coaching, you collaborate with clients to discover their answers, not yours. Clients are experts in themselves.

NBHWC competencies state that your role is not that of an educator or expert who diagnoses, advises, or tells clients what to do. Instead, in this client-centered approach you are a facilitative partner who provides the structure of the session.

ICF competencies A.2.1 and D.8.3 reiterate this focus: "Acknowledges that clients are responsible for their own choices," and "acknowledges and supports client autonomy in the design of goals, actions, and methods of accountability."

The Premature Focus Trap

What looks obvious often is not. An overweight client comes for help, and it seems reasonable to assume the focus will be on weight loss. The coach then might begin to focus the conversation on this topic while sensing the client's reluctance. Finally, the client admits, "I just quit smoking last week, and I don't know how to handle the stress of that. Could we talk about that?" A central goal for MI-style coaching would be first to focus on understanding clients' concerns and attempting to grasp their broader life situations. Prematurely choosing a focus can halt this exploration. The antidote to this trap is listening well.

The NBHWC refers to the proper timing of choosing a focus. Since you, the coach, are not the expert to decide what the focus should be, you empower the client to select what is most important, motivating, or appropriate for the moment.

ICF competency B.3.6 also stresses the importance of partnering with clients to clarify which topic to focus on: "Partners with the client to identify or reconfirm what they want to accomplish in the session."

The Labeling Trap

It could become easy to categorize clients' challenges by using labels such as "workaholic" or "food addict." The challenge with this approach is that these labels can evoke the opposite of engagement. By referring to the person or the problem with labels, you risk the client becoming less engaged and more likely to resist. The MI-consistent coach approach focuses on connecting with an active and engaged client and will, therefore, forgo using labels. Avoiding this trap will help to evoke trust and openness in a mutually respectful partnership.

As we mentioned, the NBHWC competency of trust and rapport highlights a supportive environment where the client feels accepted and safe enough to explore. ICF competency A.1.6 cautions coaches to "maintain the distinctions between coaching, consulting, psychotherapy and other support professions." In other words, the coach stays within the scope of practice and does not diagnose or label the client. These distinctions can prevent us from falling into the labeling trap.

The Blaming Trap

If clients feel blamed or if they place blame on themselves, the sessions can take a negative turn. You may often remind clients beforehand that the session will focus on the client. The emphasis should be on what is troubling them and in what ways they might decide to tackle the problem. The blaming trap could stir up defensiveness.

The NBHWC competency of client awareness, perspective shifts, and insights calls for coaches to carefully listen to how clients talk about themselves. If they are judging their own behavior, coaches are encouraged to assist clients in considering more positive self-talk. ICF competency C.7.8 says a coach "helps the client identify factors that influence current and future patterns of behavior, thinking, or emotion." This can steer the conversation toward self-responsibility and away from blame.

The Chat Trap

Chatting with a friend over a cup of coffee is one way to connect. But neither MI nor coaching are about chatting. MI's unique conversation style focuses on clients' concerns and goals, and too much chatting can divert attention away from a client's best interest. Most clients will appreciate your skill in keeping the conversation focused on their agenda and limiting time spent on extraneous pleasantries.

The NBHWC stresses that time management for each and every session is the coach's role. Coaches are expected to facilitate a conversation that allows the client to explore while also maintaining a forward-moving directional focus. This may require you to focus and refocus the conversation. The arc of the conversation may gradually build from the engaging task to client exploration, and then toward choices, goals, commitments, and plans for action. Likewise, ICF competency B.3.9 addresses this topic: "Partners with the client to manage the time and focus the session."

With the traps removed, connecting with clients becomes less like a rocky trail and more like a smooth path where momentum builds within the conversation. This engagement has a purpose; it helps clients engage with you and it can increase their motivation to change.

TWELVE ROADBLOCKS TO LISTENING

The skill of listening well is essential in all four tasks in MI. Thomas Gordon (1970) helps listeners identify what kinds of things might masquerade as listening but, in fact, become roadblocks to effective empathic listening skills. Listening well is especially important when clients are expressing their problems. Some responses, such as asking questions, sharing information, or even light joking, might be appropriate when the conversation is not centered around an issue. But these reflexive responses are not helpful within the context of the clients' expressed or assumed problem.

The 12 roadblocks to listening in the list that follows (adapted from Miller & Rollnick, 2013) tend to limit or circumvent the flow of communication away from the client and can interrupt the momentum of their exploration. The goal is to allow the client to stay on track without having to address any obstacles you may present, thereby keeping their conversation moving forward.

1. Ordering, directing, or commanding
2. Warning or threatening
3. Moralizing, telling, preaching, or lecturing
4. Advising, offering solutions, or suggesting
5. Arguing, lecturing, or persuading with logic
6. Judging, criticizing, disagreeing, or blaming
7. Labeling, shaming, or mocking
8. Interpreting, diagnosing, analyzing
9. Praising, agreeing, approving
10. Reassuring, sympathizing, consoling
11. Questioning or probing
12. Withdrawing, distracting, humoring, or changing the subject

It takes practice and effort to remove these obstacles, but once they are eliminated, your clients can more easily discover, explore, and express their ideas.

CORE SKILL: REFLECTIVE LISTENING

Accurate reflective listening, demonstrated through reflections, is the foundational skill of MI. It is at the heart of all the other MI skills. The field of coaching adopts this model of reflective listening as the foundational skill upon which all others are built. In this chapter, we introduce reflections, open questions, affirmations, and summaries. Later, we explore these skills within the context of the coaching process.

Reflective listening, also known as accurate empathy, is fundamental to all four MI tasks and to coaching as well (Rogers, 1951). This type of listening is more than being overly cordial and quietly listening to clients. It is an active way to show your understanding of clients and build engagement. Inherent in this practice is the belief that clients do best when they explore and verbalize their own thoughts and experiences. Accurate reflective listening is an invitation for clients to keep talking, exploring, and self-reflecting.

Showing empathy through reflective listening serves two purposes: You seek a deeper understanding of clients' dilemmas, and your clients gain clarity as they hear their ideas and thoughts presented back to them. You receive what is said and then offer it back to your clients as a gift in the form of reflections. You are inviting your clients to engage, and your main task is to listen accurately and reflectively.

In this initial engagement period, you will spend time exploring clients' values and goals before a direction or focus has been determined. But once the conversation shifts to focusing, evoking, or planning, you will use other types of reflections for those specific purposes. Using reflections in the other three tasks will be explored further in Chapters 5, 6, and 7.

You will need this skill before building other, more complex MI skills. As you spend time sharpening this tool in your toolbox, it will become the one you reach for throughout your coaching work. After first becoming comfortable with using reflective listening in the engaging task, you will likely find greater ease in using more complex reflections in the focusing, evoking, and planning tasks.

Reflective listening is mentioned in the NBHWC competencies. Reflections tell your clients that you hear them, and as we said earlier, they allow your clients to hear the sound of their own words, perspectives, and beliefs. Your clients will likely be engaged and inspired to learn.

Various ICF competencies indicate reflective listening in the skills of noticing, expressing, and exploring what clients say and do, which in turn facilitate clients' learning and growth.

ICF—C.6.1 "Considers the client's context, identity, environment, experiences, values, and beliefs to enhance understanding of what the client is communicating."

ICF—C.6.2 "Reflects or summarizes what the client communicated to ensure clarity and understanding."

ICF—C.6.3 "Recognizes and inquires when there is more to what the client is communicating."

ICF—C.6.4 "Notices, acknowledges, and explores the client's emotions, energy shifts, non-verbal cues, or other behaviors."

ICF—C.6.5 "Integrates the client's words, tone of voice, and body language to determine the full meaning of what is being communicated."

Attitudes Needed for Reflective Listening

How does one embark on this journey to develop the skill of reflective listening with accuracy and empathy? Miller, Rollnick, and Moyers (2019) offered a triad of attitudes in MI that, when adopted, help the practitioner develop and use the skills more easily. We adopt these in coaching.

Curiosity

First, an attitude of curiosity sends a message to clients that you are genuinely interested in their stories. Authentic curiosity about what they are saying, what they mean to say, and ways they might find a solution become the driver for reflective listening. This approach is not only effective but natural. Your beliefs about your clients' capacities and problem-solving abilities will help you uncover their inner genius.

Uncluttered Mind

Having an uncluttered mind is another essential attitude for MI practitioners (and coaches). Being overly focused on a toolbox of powerful questions and protocols or your own ideas for what is best may hinder listening intently to clients. Being uncluttered in your thinking opens the pathway to hearing and fully understanding your client's concerns.

Restraint

Curiosity and an uncluttered mind are the beginning points for listening, and then you also need restraint. Restraining your responses is both an attitude and a skill. The attitude that clients' ideas are worth hearing is reflected in your ability to limit what you say while allowing clients to carry on talking. Using pauses and silences are two ways to invite clients to keep exploring and finding possible solutions for themselves.

With these three attitudes of curiosity, an uncluttered mind, and restraint, you will most likely approach better prepared to listen carefully and follow what your clients are saying. As you engage with this mindset, reflective listening becomes more likely. The natural next step in building a stronger connection is offering reflective statements back to your clients.

The NBHWC competencies encourage building trust by using curious interest to pay attention to your clients' emotions as well as their words and behaviors. Self-management is required, especially if you feel you know what your client needs. The competencies also encourage you to refrain at times and use silence so clients can have the time and space to reflect and process. These three attitudes of mind are also reflected in the ICF competencies.

ICF—A.2 "Develops and maintains a mindset that is open, curious, flexible and client-centered."
ICF—B.5.1 "Remains focused, observant, empathetic, and responsive to the client."
ICF—B.5.2 "Demonstrates curiosity during the coaching process."
ICF—B.5.3 "Manages one's emotions to stay present with the client."
ICF—B.5.5 "Is comfortable working in a space of not knowing."
ICF—B.5.6 "Creates or allows space for silence, pause or reflection."

HOW TO FORM REFLECTIONS

In MI, there are many different types of reflections and a general sequence of skills to learn and practice. This discussion begins with simple reflections, and then we will discuss a few more complex reflections—guessing, continuing the paragraph, reflecting the underlying feeling behind what a person says, and reframing. A good beginning is to develop a habit of just listening to what a person is saying and offering it back to them as a simple reflection. (See the "Take It Further" section at the end of this chapter for practice.)

Reflective listening is a way of holding a mirror to clients' words. It is making a guess about what they expressed and allowing them to confirm—or correct—your statements. Reflections allow people to hear what they said or wanted to say. Your skillful reflective listening invites your clients to keep talking, thinking, and discovering, which is the purpose of offering reflections (Miller & Rollnick, 2023).

Hearing what people say does not always mean we understand their meaning. Their spoken words may not accurately convey what they meant, or you may not hear them correctly, or your interpretation of their words misses the mark. For this reason, it is helpful to offer an approximation—a guess—of what clients may mean.

These guesses help you draw closer and closer to understanding the client. If the guess is wrong, clients will tell you and will clarify what they mean. Reflections invite clients to explore further and spend time with their thoughts and ideas.

Nonverbal Communication

Perhaps the first step in learning to form reflections is to become a keen observer of nonverbal ways your clients communicate. You can gather important clues by attending to clients' facial expressions, body postures, eye contact, demonstration of emotions, and overall energy.

In addition to noticing and acknowledging clients' nonverbal communication, it is helpful to become conscious of the way your own presence demonstrates listening. How do you show active listening? The way you express your attention lets your clients know you are tuned in to them. Imagine clients trying to explain their thoughts and predicaments to someone who keeps shuffling papers and repeatedly glancing at a cell phone during the session. Active listening involves outwardly demonstrating your intentional focus on your client.

The NBHWC competency for active listening and presence requires listening not only to verbal information but also to nonverbal cues from coaching clients, such as expression, tone, emotions, and energy. Coaches use mindful awareness, with curiosity and nonjudgment, to notice what is happening with the client and within themselves.

Statements versus Questions

Why might you use a reflection instead of a question? Both have their proper uses in MI and coaching. The primary reason you may prefer reflections is that they are not likely to stir up reluctance. Questions can somewhat limit or determine how the conversation should go, whereas reflections open the door for further exploration.

A straightforward technique for presenting a reflection instead of a question is to intentionally turn down the voice at the end of the sentence. This is the opposite of the uplifted intonation at the end of questions. Practice saying these as a question and then as a statement.

> "Your internal saboteur is a problem?"
> "Your internal saboteur is a problem."
> "You cannot imagine giving up wine?"
> "You can't imagine giving up wine."

An additional technique is to first think about the question you may have in your mind, then remove the question words and the inflection at the end.

CLIENT: I can't imagine giving up wine.

COACH: [The question in your mind.] Do you mean you have not tried to quit drinking wine?

COACH: [The reflection spoken to the client.] You have not tried to quit drinking wine.

SIMPLE REFLECTIONS

A simple reflection is the practice of repeating one or more words clients say or slightly rephrasing their words without adding much to them. At times, nothing more is required to keep the dialogue going. As you develop this skill, a simple reflection is a place to begin, however, the caution is to notice if the conversation becomes stagnant and fails to advance, which may mean you may have used too many simple reflections. For this reason, incorporating more complex reflections can elicit further conversation and, thus, more understanding. Additionally, with careful listening, you will also be able to detect if too many wrong guesses have strained the dialogue.

CLIENT: I'm not a very patient person.

COACH: You're not a very patient person. [*Simple reflection, restating.*]

COACH: You're less patient than you want to be. [*A more complex reflection of the possible meaning.*]

COMPLEX REFLECTIONS

A complex reflection adds depth to the clients' words, whether it infers meaning or makes a guess to continue the flow of the paragraph. It is as if you wave a flag in the path, signaling clients to keep moving forward. This skill of offering complex reflections takes practice but is worth the effort, since the result is greater communication and understanding. Here are four types of complex reflections: guessing, continuing the paragraph, reflecting underlying feeling, and reframing. See Chapter 7 for a discussion of double-sided reflections.

Guessing

Offering complex reflections might be viewed as guessing because, as we mentioned, we cannot be certain about the meaning of someone else's words. You might be correct or somewhat wrong, but making a guess signals to clients that you are attempting to understand their accurate meaning.

Guessing is different than assuming. Making assumptions is discouraged, since it may imply bias toward your perspective rather than your clients' expertise in their own lives.

Complex reflections are dynamic; the energy of the reflection nudges to the front what otherwise might have been unspoken. In taking a risk by guessing, you will find either a correction or a confirmation. If you missed the mark, this is not a problem, and this will likely only lead you to become more accurate with follow-up reflections. If you were correct, or somewhat correct, the client will let you know, often with an aha confirmation: "Yes, that is exactly what I meant!" To be heard and understood in this way is a profoundly satisfying experience for most people. When you guess as a coach, offering it as a statement rather than a question will provide the opportunity to check your guesses.

Continuing the Paragraph

Another type of complex reflection is continuing the paragraph. According to Miller and Rollnick (2023), continuing the paragraph moves the conversation forward by making a gentle prompting about what might be said next. Again, if your guess is wrong, the person will probably be happy to elaborate and help your understanding. This type of reflection creates momentum and opens the door for hearing what clients might not have verbalized. You are keeping the conversation in motion.

Coaching Sample: Continuing the Paragraph Reflection in Coaching

CLIENT: I started the week off right and was really motivated to get that sweatshirt made like I planned to do, but something else came up that ended up being even better.

COACH: You felt comfortable adjusting your plans.

CLIENT: Right, I've been tied to my schedule and too hard on myself if I don't follow through on plans. When I remembered it was Valentine's Day this week, I had a sudden inspiration to make a vintage hoodie for my boyfriend instead of the other project I had on my schedule.

COACH: This project seemed more important to you, so you went for it.

CLIENT: I was ready to go on my first plan, but once I started sketching this new thing, I had the "flow" we talked about. I worked for seven straight hours on this, and it didn't even feel like work.

COACH: Instead of being restricted by your schedule, you allowed your passion for this project to drive you forward into action.

CLIENT: Right! I've been too rigid and too afraid to trust my artistic visions. That kept me from being creative.

COACH: You feel that rigidity stops your creative flow, and you like being in charge of your schedule.

CLIENT: It feels like a relief not to have guilt about being artistic and just going with the flow. Instead of writing what my next project should be for this week's goal, I may just block off time for "creative work." This feels much more like my style.

Notice how the coach does not insert roadblocks but gives reflections that invite the client to keep exploring. For effect, try reading the above paragraph without the coach's comments and notice the sense of continuity.

Reflecting Underlying Feeling

Listening on a deeper level sometimes uncovers clients' feelings or emotions behind the words. These unstated emotions are important and, when surfaced, can help to generate clients' insights and spark ideas for change (Miller et al., 2019). Listening like this is about paying attention to the emotional state of the other.

When using this type of reflection, you use the MI skill (discussed earlier) of noticing nonverbal communication to gather cues from the client. Bringing these feelings and emotions to the surface may spark clients' insights and increase their capacity for change.

The NBHWC competencies encourage coaches to begin sessions by asking clients to assess their "state." Coaches attend to clients' moods, emotions, and presence and ask clients to describe these when appropriate. Coaches notice and spotlight any positive shifts in the clients' energy or emotions as a way to support change. With this awareness, coaches encourage positive acceptance of emotions in exchange for any self-criticism that discourages insight. This practice demonstrates empathy and fosters self-compassion.

There is a clear parallel between MI and the NBHWC in terms of the emphasis on reflections, as stated in the related competency overview. The NBHWC coach competencies prioritize reflections as a key component of active listening, which helps engage the client and facilitate learning. These competencies outline various types of MI reflections, including simple, complex, double-sided, reflecting feelings and meaning, and summaries.

ICF—A.2.5 "Uses awareness of self and one's intuition to benefit clients."

ICF—B.4.5 "Acknowledges and supports the client's expression of feelings, perceptions, concerns, beliefs, and suggestions."

ICF—B.4.4 "Demonstrates confidence in working with strong client emotions during the coaching process."

ICF—C.6.3 "Recognizes and inquires when there is more to what the client is communicating."

ICF—C.6.5 "Integrates the client's words, tone of voice and body language to determine the full meaning of what is being communicated."

ICF—C.6.6 "Notices trends in the client's behaviors and emotions across sessions to discern themes and patterns."

ICF—C.7.11 "Shares observations, insights and feelings, without attachment, that have the potential to create new learning for the client."

Coaching Sample: Reflection of Underlying Feeling

COACH: You seem a bit troubled today.

CLIENT: I am. I read over the diet my doctor gave me, and there's a lot to it. I didn't know it would be so involved and that I would have to give up so many of my favorite foods.

COACH: You feel surprised and disappointed about the diet. [*A guess.*]

CLIENT: Well, maybe not so much disappointed, but for sure I'm surprised. My husband won't do this diet, so I'll have to cook for him, my kids, and me, and it's too much. [*Client clarifies.*]

COACH: It's overwhelming to follow the diet if you have to make two different meals for yourself and your family. [*Reflects underlying feelings.*]

CLIENT: Well, now that I think about it, it's not that complicated. I mean, I was surprised and even a little overwhelmed. But I think I can do it. It'll be hard, but at least now I know what I'll need to prepare for next week. [*This indicates the coach is closer to understanding the dilemma.*]

COACH: Even though this is hard for you, you feel confident this is something you can do.

CLIENT: That's right, I can figure this out.

The coach made a guess, which was only partially correct. As the client clarifies their feelings, they explore more about how they might approach this challenge.

Reframing

When clients view things through a limited or negative lens, you can offer reflections to reframe or shine a more positive light to heighten clients' self-awareness and shift perspectives. At other times, when clients see things in a somewhat overly optimistic light, reframing might allow them to see the possible downside of things if that is needed. In reframing, you take what the person says that may have a negative (or positive) meaning and offer a different interpretation.

Reframing is mentioned in the NBHWC competencies of client awareness, perspective shifts, and insights. Coaches are encouraged to reflect on the clients' views and ask open-ended questions to foster self-awareness and new perspectives. NBHWC suggests offering an alternative and more positive perspective, since this is more likely to inspire motivation and forward progress. NBHWC proposes that coaches listen for any negative self-talk or judgment and help clients reframe perspectives to consider more positive self-talk. The ICF also directs coaches to support reframing.

> ICF—C.7.10 "Supports the client in reframing perspectives."
> ICF—D.8.7 "Celebrates the client's progress and successes."

Coaching Sample: Reframing Reflections

CLIENT: I failed this week. I planned to be 100% alcohol-free, but it was my friend's birthday, so we went out for dinner, and I had a glass of dry red wine. I didn't have any alcohol the rest of the week, and I could tell I had less brain fog without the booze.

COACH: You allowed yourself to celebrate with your friend and you made a choice to have a low-sugar wine option. Your choice was a better one than you have made in the past. That's a win!

Using reflections in an MI-consistent conversation within a coaching session will take intentional practice and self-review. Another way to improve is to receive feedback from peers who review recorded sessions and then report on the chosen target, such as the number and type of reflections used during the session. We elaborate on this practice in Chapter 15.

IMPROVING ACTIVE REFLECTIVE LISTENING

Below is a list of ways you could improve reflective listening in the four tasks.

In the Engaging Task

1. Fewer words are preferred. Be brief and to the point.
2. Make one guess, keep it simple.
3. Remember the purpose: understand your client's dilemma, no specific direction yet.
4. Remember the plan: convey your understanding back to the client.
5. Most of your responses should be reflective-listening statements.
6. Use reflections to follow up on your open questions.
7. Maintain the attitudes of curiosity, clarity of mind, and restraint.
8. Avoid the question/answer trap by asking more questions than reflections, as this may spark defensiveness.

In the Evoking Task

1. Reflections in the evoking part elicit self-awareness, learning, and insight and will be used to accelerate forward movement toward change.

In All Four Tasks

1. Offer at least half of your responses as reflections.
2. Aim for twice as many reflections as questions.

Coaching Sample: Reflective Listening in Engaging, in an Early Session

COACH: You've come here to work on your stress. Tell me more about that.

CLIENT: Yea, I'm stressed over everything. Work is crazy now with the turnovers, and I can't turn off my brain when I get home. It's affecting how I deal with the kids. I mean, they have their own issues when they get home from school, too, and I need to be emotionally available for them. Being stressed makes it hard to pay attention to their needs, and then I feel guilty and have more stress.

COACH: You want to be emotionally available for your kids, and your stress keeps you from that.

[*A simple reflection. The coach is curious to explore the client's possible source of motivation for change, so this simple reflection invites the client to keep talking.*]

CLIENT: That's true; it's getting in the way. I remember feeling that my mother was too busy with her own life to pay attention to me. I don't want that for my kids, but I can't manage everything at once.

COACH: You sound regretful that you missed out on your mother's attention. And you want something better for your kids. [*Reflecting feeling, and affirming the client's positive strengths and qualities.*]

CLIENT: That's right! It makes me sad. I've told myself I wouldn't do that to my own kids, but I'm covered up with stress and acting like my mother, and my anxiety is impacting my relationship with my spouse, too. We argue a lot lately, and that wouldn't happen if I could chill out a little more. I don't know what to do.

COACH: On the one hand, you want to show love to your kids and spouse, and be there for them, and on the other hand, you are too stressed to care for them the way you want to.

[*Complex reflection of the client's ambivalence. This indicates that the coach is listening and seeking to understand the client's dilemma. Accurate empathy.*]

CLIENT: Right! It sounds crazy, doesn't it? I want to change so my kids can have a different experience than I had growing up. [*The coach's complex reflection prompted increased awareness.*]

COACH: You know what you want for your family, and you can't care for them in the way you'd like. Once you manage your stress, you'll be emotionally available to be the type of mother and spouse you want to be. [*Complex reflection.*]

The coach has not asked questions yet, but the series of reflections and a short summary opened the door for the client to keep exploring. These reflections helped the coach uncover more details and further understand the client's key issues. The coach is building a relationship of trust where the client can share without fear of judgment or disapproval.

CORE SKILL: OPEN QUESTIONS

The skill of asking open questions helps you better engage and understand clients, focus the direction of the conversation, evoke their motivation, and plan for change. In contrast, closed questions are answered with a "yes" or "no" and are designed to gather specific information. Collecting client information from a checklist of fact-gathering questions might seem efficient at first glance but does little to allow clients the opportunity to ponder and expand on their thoughts. If one seeks quick information, a checklist might suffice. However, neither MI nor coaching focus primarily on that type of client information. Instead, the goal of asking open questions is to understand the person's perspective better while also continuing to build a strong partnership that opens the door for client exploration and discovery.

Open questions can elicit more information than a written intake assessment. However, asking a series of even the most well-formed open questions could potentially limit responses and inadvertently stifle clients' exploration. Instead, using a mix of open questions and reflective statements invites clients to continue their discovery. For this reason, skillful coaches use both. Effective MI practice prefers a ratio of two reflections for every question (Miller & Rollnick, 2023). For coaches, we suggest a ratio of at least one reflection for every question. See Table 4.1 for a sample of closed versus open questions.

Open questions are encouraged in the NBHWC competency focused on expanding the conversation. Curious questions evoke deeper thinking and self-reflection and help expand possibilities. "What" or "How" open questions encourage client exploration and can be used to emphasize strengths, values, and further learning. These types of questions can foster a broader perspective and help clients discover interconnections in their lives. ICF competency C.7.4 also emphasizes the power of open questions: "Asks questions that help the client explore beyond current thinking."

Coaching Sample: Open-Ended Questions in the Engaging Task

COACH: What brings you to coaching?

CLIENT: I'm having trouble with work–life balance.

TABLE 4.1. Open versus Closed Questions

Closed questions	Open questions
• Did you complete all your time management goals this week?	• What did you accomplish since our last session that you are pleased with?
• Did you send out your resume?	• What was it like to send out your resume?
• Is your spouse a good support for you?	• What kind of support might you need?
• Are you going to set a goal around your stress management?	• What do you need to consider around your goal of managing stress?
• Didn't the doctor tell you to stop smoking?	• How would it improve your life if you stopped smoking?
• Would you like to talk about how to cut back on sugar or discuss your use of alcohol to relieve stress? *(Giving options is a form of closed questions that limit clients' responses.)*	• Which of the topics you mentioned feels more important for our work today?

COACH: What about finding balance do you find most challenging? [*Open question.*]

CLIENT: I get out of balance when I'm doing what I'm passionate about—my art—and then I don't care about my basic needs, like eating and sleeping well.

COACH: Your passion motivates you to work hard. [*Complex reflection.*]

CLIENT: That's true. I love it, but I'm afraid of where it's leading me. I don't like how I get so burned out.

COACH: Something has given you a warning here, and you're listening to the signals. What are some ways that you feel imbalanced? [*Open question.*]

CLIENT: I got so one-sided last year on the work that I neglected my own personal needs. I want to work as an artist without losing myself along the way, but I haven't succeeded.

COACH: Having balance is an important part of your happiness. [*Complex reflection.*]

The coach uses both open questions and reflective statements to elicit more information in this early session.

CORE SKILL: AFFIRMATIONS

Affirming clients is a way of noticing and commenting on their inherent worth and acknowledging their unique strengths, efforts, and better qualities. Developing this habit of mind requires intentionally seeking out the client's positive side. Criticism and judgment are poor motivators, but authentic affirmations inspire and motivate.

When learning how to use affirmations, it is helpful to recall the attitudes we explored in the discussion of the MI spirit and the coach approach. Accepting people for who they are, regardless of what predicament they are in, is what is meant by "acceptance." This approach encourages you to seek out, emphasize, and celebrate the positive aspects of individuals. The opposite is the "fixing reflex," the desire to fix what is wrong with people (Miller & Rollnick, 2023).

Affirmations are used in slightly different ways in each task, depending on their purpose. In engaging, you seek to build the relationship, demonstrate empathy, and show an understanding of the client's challenges.

How do you use and develop this skill? Like MI practitioners, you will first focus on the client's positive aspects, taking care to avoid the roadblock of giving praise (Gordon, 1970). Praising your client may imply assumed superiority as if you were in the position to assign value to their actions. Instead of using "I" in statements such as, "I am proud of your good effort," try substituting the word "you" (Miller & Rollnick, 2023). "You gave it good effort this week, even though you still ate some cake."

Another way to affirm clients is to highlight a personal strength or skill, especially when they are discouraged and feel as if they failed.

"I messed up again this week. I ate a few bites of cake."

"You ate some cake, but you didn't eat the whole piece! You used your self-regulation this week and made progress!"

In addition to spotlighting a specific skill, affirmations may also demonstrate your genuine appreciation of your clients: "You're a creative problem-solver."

Affirmations are a part of the NBHWC competency that aims to increase positive psychological resources. Affirming clients' self-worth and efforts can help develop these positive resources by exploring meaning and reflecting on their positive emotions. Focusing on these positive resources (positive psychology) can enhance clients' ability to think creatively and strategically, remain open-minded, act with resilience, and make meaningful connections.

The NBHWC competencies call for exploring, developing, and affirming what is good about your clients. This includes their skills, progress, positive traits, insights, and learning, along with values, self-worth and acceptance, optimism, and resilience. This important MI skill of offering affirmations is also a part of the ICF competencies.

ICF—B.4.3 "Acknowledges and respects the client's unique talents, insights, and work in the coaching process."

ICF—C.7.6 "Notices what is working to enhance client progress."

ICF—D.8.4 "Supports the client in identifying potential results or learning from identified action steps."

ICF—D.8.6 "Partners with the client to summarize learning and insight within or between sessions."

ICF—D.8.7 "Celebrates the client's progress and successes."

CORE SKILL: SUMMARIES

Summaries are types of longer reflections. In the engaging and focusing tasks, summaries show that you paid attention to your clients and valued what they said. Later, in the evoking task, summaries collect the clients' reasons and arguments for change (change talk) in order to highlight and influence the conversation toward forward progress. Summaries in the planning task pull together motivations and plans for change.

Summaries are used in the engaging task to illuminate the clients' stories and invite them to continue exploring. Miller and Rollnick (2023) referred to this practice with a vivid analogy of collecting the bits of the client's story as if they were cut flowers, which are then arranged into a beautiful bouquet and presented back to the client as a gift.

It can also be helpful to offer shorter summaries throughout the conversation to let clients hear what they said while paving the way for them to continue. (A smaller collection of flowers is what florists call a posy.) You offer back a nice posy of the seemingly unrelated statements the person shared. But what types of things do you offer in the engaging task? The type of summary depends on your purpose.

Collecting Summary

A *collecting summary* could invite your client to consider possibilities. "What things would be different for you if you lived your best life a year from now?" After hearing a few of the client's ideas, you would collect this as a summary. These collecting summaries tend to orient the conversation while also communicating that you are tracking along with them.

> "So far, you can imagine being healthy enough to play with your daughter because you're at a healthy weight. You would have more time to be with your family if you stopped working 60 hours a week. You would enjoy being outside, riding a bike, or even running again. What else can you imagine?"

Linking Summary

A *linking summary* is used when you want to connect what clients may have said in an earlier session with what they are saying now.

> "Last week, you felt you hadn't reflected on what might sabotage your progress. And today, you discovered more about yourself because you started journaling your thoughts every day."

Transitional Summary

The third type of summary is one you might use when you want to move on to something else in the session. These *transitional* summaries pull things together that have been important so far in the conversation and bridge them to what may come next.

> "You want to work on building confidence, and before we talk about that, let's make sure I've heard you correctly so far. You were confident when things were going well with your art. Something changed, your life shifted out of balance, and you stopped taking care of yourself. You're a bit discouraged, and this has you frozen right now. You're hesitant to get started, even though you know how much potential you have."

In all these summaries, clients are invited to take a bird's-eye view of what they said and gaze at their own thoughts. This perspective often invites powerful insights, and clients are stirred to broaden their self-awareness and reflection. This intentional and empathic listening is a rare gift, one that is not always part of everyday conversations. The NBHWC competencies refer to summaries as a skill in the topic of reflections. The ICF-related competencies also include summaries.

ICF—C.6.2 "Reflects or summarizes what the client communicated to ensure clarity and understanding."

ICF—D.8.6 "Partners with the client to summarize learning and insight within or between sessions."

Coaching Sample: A Summary in the Engaging Task

CLIENT: I got a text message from a former friend who treated me poorly in the past. She wanted to start our friendship again, but the last time we spoke, she was disrespectful and rude. I was clear and honest about my boundaries and how I needed to be treated, and she didn't like that. I said I couldn't be around that negative energy. I didn't blame her, I just communicated what wasn't working for me in our friendship.

COACH: Your communication was honest and mature. You used your wisdom to recognize that she was not coming from an equal place in your relationship. You felt taken advantage of, but you stood up for yourself and set your boundaries with love and fairness. You stayed in integrity with yourself then, and you remain in integrity now.

In this example, the coach chooses to reflect the positive statements of the client. The coach offers a summary focusing on the client's strengths, indicating that the coach is listening at a deeper level without judgment or bias.

Take It Further

Work with a partner in your learning community to reflect on and answer the following questions.

1. How are empowerment and autonomy promoted in the engaging task? (See the NBHWC competencies that focus on the client-centered relationship and the client's freedom of choice and autonomy and ICF D.8, etc.).
2. What are the three suggested attitudes needed for reflective listening? Find the NBHWC competencies that focus on trust and rapport, active listening and presence, and the ICF competencies (A.2, B.5.1–B.5.6) to explain.
3. Explain the purpose of offering reflections. Which NBHWC and ICF competencies support this?
   a. Create examples of complex reflections, such as continuing the paragraph, guessing, reflecting underlying meanings or feelings, and reframing.
4. Beside each coach statement, write the letter indicating which core skill is demonstrated: open question, affirmation, reflection, or summary (OARS).
   a. "What about this job makes you anxious?" ______
   b. "You applied a lot of concentrated effort to be patient with your son." ______
   c. "You have tried many strategies already, and yet you don't feel successful." ______
   d. "So far, the lack of sleep is the most pressing issue, and you are also concerned about setting boundaries at work." ______
5. Read the definitions below and label each as either an open question, an affirmation, a reflection, or a summary (OARS).
   a. Requires more than a "yes" or "no" answer or a limited amount of information. ______
   b. Links the client's statements together as either a large bouquet or a small posy. ______
   c. Makes a guess about the client's meaning of the words. ______
   d. Acknowledges client's strength, effort, value, successes, or goals. ______
   e. Inspires and shows empathy and understanding of client's dilemmas. ______
   f. Demonstrates curiosity and genuine interest in the client. ______

Chapter 5

The Focusing Task

Your clients are sitting in front of you because they want to move from their current state to a better one; they want to change and grow. You are headed somewhere with the client. The task of focusing gives you a context and structure for guiding the conversation—and the client—forward. Focusing is finding and clarifying the goal or goals toward which you and the client will work together. It is the bridge for moving forward.

COACHING DISTINCTIONS

There are several critical differences between coaches and therapists, counselors, or mentors. As a coach, you are not primarily concerned with knowledge exchange or treating matters related to mental health. Your clients are not seeking treatment to eliminate psychological problems or dysfunctions. Your job is not to treat, repair, or dispense your expert advice. However, some coaching skills overlap with counseling, such as focusing on the relationship, engaging with the clients, and guiding a forward-moving conversation. As we mentioned, coaching and counseling with MI both focus on building a relationship of trust and compassion.

We have shown that MI overlaps with coaching and the coach approach. However, there is an important distinction to be made between coaching and the general model of treatment. This might be best illustrated in the illness–wellness continuum created by Dr. John Travis and explained by Wellness Associates (2018).

Figure 5.1 is a simple illustration that shows the paradigm of helping clients change and grow toward an ideal self and life. We view coaching as existing on this continuum, where therapy and treatment are on one end. The scope of coaching overlaps with that of therapy, and a search for a clear distinction has been a topic of debate as the coaching field continues to develop (Sime & Jacob, 2018).

Disease or disorder is on the left end of the illness–wellness continuum. The diagram depicts how therapeutic interventions use a treatment model, moving persons from the left to the neutral point, where neither illness nor high-level wellness is present. Coaches operate from this neutral point, helping people move progressively to the right, which indicates a life of flourishing and well-being. From the neutral point, people can move rightward as they become more aware and informed, and as they adopt and maintain new lifestyle behaviors.

In your work, you might uncover clients' early warning signs of illness, trauma, or a clinical disorder during the engaging and focusing tasks. You may hear signs of disease or remnants of unresolved conditions that manifest as forms of physical, mental, or emotional maladaptive patterns. These patterns warrant specialized treatment and a possible referral to a trained therapist. While engaging with your client, you may have uncovered something outside your scope of practice, and this can be viewed as one positive outcome of active listening in the focusing task. Even if clients are referred to a clinician, it is not uncommon for them to work with a coach simultaneously.

Suppose clients are hesitant to seek therapy but want to receive coaching. In that case, you may choose to continue coaching while creating a safe environment, respecting the client's autonomy, and supporting their self-compassion. These clients may eventually be ready to seek therapy when they feel safe and supported.

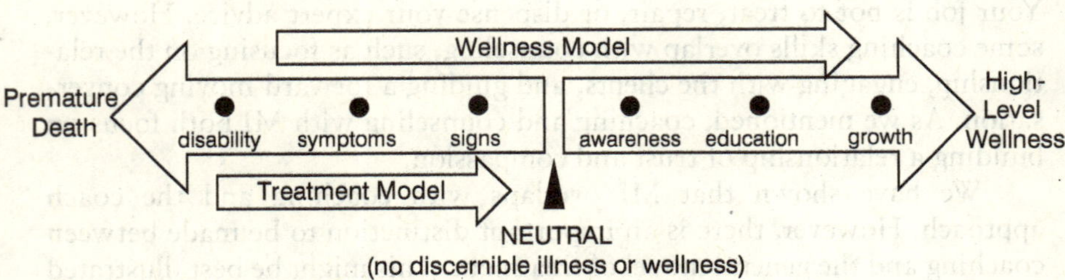

FIGURE 5.1. The illness–wellness continuum.

Coaching Sample: A Coach Conversation Where a Referral Is Needed

COACH: What did you accomplish last week that you're pleased with?

CLIENT: Nothing. I've been sleeping too much, and I want to eat better, but I don't feel like cooking.

COACH: This is unusual for you. [*Reflect meaning.*]

CLIENT: Yeah, I used to care more about things than I do now.

COACH: You suspect something isn't quite right. [*A guess.*]

CLIENT: I don't know what it is, but I'm just going through the motions. I'm sad all the time.

COACH: Your sleeping has changed, and you're not enjoying life right now, and being sad feels constant. [*Coach offers a summary reflection and recognizes some "red flags."*]

(*Client nods.*)

I understand. This must be pretty tough, especially as you're trying to improve your stress management. How long do you think you've felt like this? [*Empathy, and open question.*]

CLIENT: For about 6 weeks or so before I came to you for coaching.

COACH: You've noticed changes in your mood that we don't want to ignore, which shows an awareness on your part. The symptoms you're describing need to be shared with your medical professional. Would you be interested in a referral to a mental health therapist that I've referred clients to in the past? [*Empathy, referral, and closed question used appropriately.*]

CLIENT: That's probably a good idea. But I'd like to stay with you for coaching if that's all right.

COACH: Sure, as long as it doesn't interfere with your work with the therapist and as long as you feel you're getting value out of coaching.

AGREEMENTS AND FOCUS

Coaches who adhere to standards from the ICF and the NBHWC prioritize the task of focusing in the coaching relationship. Focusing occurs both in the initial sessions as you develop a relationship with your client, and also as you assume responsibility for maintaining the focus over the course of your work with the client.

ICF uses the term "agreements," which is interchangeable with the term "focus" found in the NBHWC documents. In the ICF competencies, you and the client make agreements about the process and parameters of the coaching relationship and the overall coaching arrangement. You also make specific agreements about the client's desired outcomes for the coaching engagement as well as the focus (goals) for individual sessions.

The NBHWC presents "focus" in two parts. First, you allow time for clients to explore a broader focus and clarify their larger vision, values, purpose, and priorities. Invite them to choose a priority focus in an area related to and inspired by this larger vision or long-term goal. Second, you ask them to select the focus for each session. Clients view their current state compared to their optimal vision, and the discrepancy between those two—the gap—becomes the launchpad for going forward. (See the NBHWC and ICF core competencies at *www.guilford.com/lanier-materials*.)

The term "agreements" implies a collaborative design. The NBHWC competencies emphasize that the coach is not the "expert" who chooses the focus for the client but instead the coach empowers the client to select an area for themselves that feels important, motivating, or timely.

This competency implies a hierarchy of goals, where long- and short-term goals are supported by a series of strategic action steps toward those goals. Both sets of standards highlight the role of collaboration in choosing a focus aligned with the client's desires, needs, and personal choices. In MI-consistent coaching, the client's autonomy for selecting a focus is kept foremost.

MOTIVATION IN THE FOCUSING TASK

Relevant Concepts and Theories

How can you facilitate your clients' movements toward change? What relevant behavior change theories and discoveries inform your efforts to ignite motivation and forward momentum? MI is founded on certain ideas about motivation, and the field of coaching builds upon those ideas. Here, we provide an overview of a few fundamental theories, and then we suggest some practical applications for your practice.

If change were as straightforward as finding and closing the gap between behavior and values, the current state, and the ideal future, coaches might not be needed. But we observe from human experience that change is not usually that simple. For some, becoming aware of this gap is the only motivation needed to get things moving. For example, a doctor warns that smoking has damaged a person's lungs, and the person quits cold turkey. But for others, even a dire warning fails to spark a change, much less sustain it for the long term.

Dr. Daniella Steyn assumed that her patients would make necessary lifestyle changes after receiving a prescription or protocol from her. The reality is that patient compliance is sometimes minimal, especially where lifestyle behaviors are concerned: "I was surprised that patients who seemed motivated have gone to the trouble to find me, have made an appointment, paid money, and submitted to extensive testing, but fail to follow through with the recommendations I give them" (Steyn, 2022). Something was missing. This discovery prompted Dr. Steyn to employ health and wellness coaches to help patients move toward compliance and ultimately toward their ideal selves and thriving lives.

Professional coaches may not have the same training and education as therapists, but a foundational understanding of how people change can help coaches adapt and "dance in the moment" in service of clients' varied needs. Some clients are ready and confident and only need a plan of action. At the other extreme are those less ready, maybe discouraged, demotivated, or reluctant to follow a third party's recommendation. You will personalize your service by using what best suits your clients. These theories are integrated into MI and can become the backbone of the strategies in your coaching toolbox. They can provide the "why" for what you do.

Self-Determination Theory

In addition to the Rogerian client-centered approach that we mentioned, MI is consistent with Deci and Ryan's self-determination theory (SDT), especially because of SDT's premise that motivation and personal autonomy are critical issues in behavior change. MI's proposition that clients will decide for themselves whether to change is an echo of SDT. People already possess this power, and it is something that cannot be taken away. The hallmark lesson of the SDT model is that a disengaged client predicts poor long-term success in goal attainment. According to SDT, lasting change most likely occurs when clients are actively engaged and invested in change (Ryan & Deci, 2008).

Clients who have intrinsic motivation, confidence about new behaviors, and other people to support and encourage them are more likely to have successful and long-term change. Furthermore, people progress more readily when the desired change aligns with their personal beliefs and values. Individuals are motivated by personal factors and thrive best when the three basic psychological needs are met: autonomy, competence, and relatedness.

MI's core elements echo these needs by emphasizing clients' internal motivation (autonomy), working together with the client on the successful attainment of goals (competence), and the compassionate relationship that supports growth (relatedness). Motivation in SDT is something to develop within the process of the therapeutic (and coaching) setting, as opposed to being a prerequisite (Spence & Oades, 2011). Like in MI, based on SDT, coaches evoke people's intrinsic motivation for change, and this is accomplished with an MI-consistent conversational approach.

SDT in Coaching

All people need to feel in charge of their lives. They need to feel confident and effective, and above all, they need to feel connected to others (who support their autonomy). These are vital to fuel motivation for change. Self-regulation can occur when the client's social and physical environment supports and meets those three needs. The coaching relationship can assist in the satisfaction of those needs. We do not suggest that the coaching relationship can meet those needs entirely. Still, coaching can provide a container in which the conversation enhances the satisfaction of those needs (Spence & Oades, 2011). What can a coach do to help foster this kind of environment? Notice the overtones of MI in the list below.

- Support autonomy by emphasizing clients' core values, desires, and choices.
- Support competence (self-efficacy for the chosen task) by acknowledging clients' strengths, resources, and capabilities.
- Support relatedness by demonstrating compassion, honesty, and trust. Even more specifically, you can use the MI skills of empathy, reflective listening, and affirming strengths and efforts, which have the potential to enliven human flourishing.

The focusing task is the beginning of discovering what motivates your clients. It is a process of connecting their long- and short-term goals to larger core values, purpose, and vision. To achieve lasting change, it is more effective to choose goals that are created autonomously and driven by intrinsic motivation. Social support, important in identifying what motivates people, is also found—among other places—in the coach–client relationship (O'Hara, 2017).

Self-Efficacy Theory

According to Albert Bandura (1997), self-efficacy, a component of social cognitive theory (SCT), is a strong predictor of success in making changes (Bandura & Cervone, 1983). Self-efficacy defines one's hope about the ability to reach specific goals, which determines both the amount of effort and the time spent on sustained work toward the goal. Bandura's positive message is that people possess the capacity to affect their internal and external barriers to behavior change. Competence results from the experience of success, and confidence is the fruit of that success and potential future achievements. Confidence includes both the perception of how important a change is and the perceived assurance that the person is capable of making the change. If clients make better choices, this leads to more success and, in turn, results in greater confidence for the following action. The cycle is self-perpetuating (Moore et al., 2016).

MI emphasizes building self-efficacy to support internal motivation. As a coach, you foster self-efficacy by allowing clients to choose and work toward goals tied to their core values and what is important to them.

Self-Efficacy Theory in Coaching

The focusing task is the place to begin listening for and building self-efficacy. In searching for an area of focus or a destination, you will listen for or inquire directly about each client's level of confidence around specific challenges. For those lacking hope, stirring up their energy to change may take concerted effort. The good news is that MI-consistent coaching offers a relationship within which the seeds of hope begin to grow. The first skill is listening. The germination of hope can be in the engagement, the relationship, and the resulting conversation that fosters competence.

Some clients are sponsored or incentivized to receive coaching, while others come to it because they have not yet achieved their personal or professional desired growth. Some may be a bit overwhelmed with multiple things to change, and they want help deciding where to start. To foster your clients' sense of competence and confidence to change, you can skillfully use MI-consistent conversations to build their confidence. (The specific skill of evoking will be explored in depth in Chapter 6.)

A Short List of Ways to Foster Self-Efficacy in the Focusing Task

- Listen for and use open questions to inquire about confidence.
- Resist the urge to rush toward goal setting. Spend time evoking confidence.
- Highlight and affirm strengths rather than weaknesses.
- Assist clients in recognizing past successes, small accomplishments, and learnings.
- Help clients positively reframe their narratives and experiences.
- Invite clients' self-awareness and support them in finding possibilities for growth.
- Invite clients to create a compelling, forward-focused, detailed, and expansive vision of their ideal self and future.
- Support clients in choosing role models of their desired behavior, someone they can relate to.

Act on the belief that clients are naturally "creative, resourceful, and whole" (Kimsey-House et al., 2018) and convey that they can—with the proper support—use their ability to act as positive change agents in their lives. Self-beliefs are potent tools that can be used to exercise self-control "over their thoughts, feelings, and actions; what people think, believe, and feel affects how they behave" (Bandura, 2008).

Working Alliance Theory

The quality of the working alliance between practitioner and client predicts outcome. This finding is consistent in the research across a broad spectrum of treatment contexts (Horvath et al., 2011). As discussed earlier, the MI spirit (the coaches' CAPE) aids in forging a robust, empathic relationship between practitioner and client. This warm, compassionate relationship is considered one of the necessary contributing factors in a "working alliance." The other key component is having clear, shared goals and agreement on the tasks for achieving the goals. When you and clients behave in a collaborative process of discussing and agreeing upon goals, this working alliance itself becomes therapeutic (Tryon & Winograd, 2011). The result is better outcomes for the client.

The Working Alliance in Coaching

The coaching profession models its practice on these findings. The ICF and NBHWC competencies reverberate this message in co-creating goals, partnering to find focus, and doing so in an atmosphere of trust and safety.

Taking a cue from the research, this working alliance is best built very early in the coaching engagement. The entry point is the engaging task but continues as a vital component during the focusing task as you and the client work collaboratively to find a direction. Building on lessons from the study and practice of MI, here are a few practical ways that you can create a strong working alliance in the focusing task.

- Engage clients in discussing topics important to them, ones that hold value.
- Use reflective listening so that clients feel understood.
- Collaborate—invite clients to choose the focus and offer your ideas (with permission) in a shared discovery or brainstorming activity.
- Emphasize mutual agreement of the focus.
- Gain clarity on the focus, allowing clients to summarize or refine the focus.
- Activate client engagement by discussing concerns or feelings around the focus.
- Your role is to focus and refocus the conversations to stay on course. You do this in a way that respects each client's autonomy.
- Remain flexible and attentive, checking periodically to see if a client's focus has been modified or needs clarification.

The Stages of Change

Stages of change is part of the transtheoretical model (TTM) that emerged concurrent to the development of MI and is one way to view the structure of behavior change. As noted in Chapter 2, this influential model for helping people change appeared in the 1980s as a collection of the common components of primary therapies about change. Prochaska and colleagues (1992) described five somewhat controllable and predictable stages that people typically pass through when making a change: precontemplation (no interest in making changes), contemplation (thinking about changing), preparation (preparing for change), action (recently taking steps to change), and then maintenance (sustaining change over time). Having both options for processes and techniques that can be used during each stage helps clients prepare for a change and lets the helping practitioner know how to frame the conversation and support growth.

Most other models are designed to help clients in the "I'm ready" stage of change. MI emerged partly to answer the question about how to help clients who are in the less ready stage, those who say "I can't" or "I won't" or are in the "I'm thinking about it" stage, those clients who are more ambivalent about change. Once again, the first MI skill is deep, reflective listening while giving clients space to explore and express their perspectives. Being knowledgeable about the stages of change will help you use the most effective method in each stage to help clients move forward to the next stage.

As noted in Chapter 2, some people assume that MI is only applicable in the coaching process until the client's ambivalence has been resolved. They argue that MI is no longer needed once a person is in the planning and action stage. We believe this is a misunderstanding of MI, and our aim is to demonstrate the integration of MI throughout the entire coaching process, from beginning to end. It is a continual golden thread that is woven through the entire tapestry of coaching.

Coaching with the Transtheoretical Model

Later, in Chapter 6 and throughout the rest of this book, we dive into the specific MI strategies that you might use to help clients in each stage. Here are a few essential principles of change to keep in mind in the focusing task.

- *Normalize the spiral process of change and allow clients to understand their own stage of change.* When clients understand the stages and the most helpful processes within each stage, they gain more control over the cycle of change and move more quickly through each stage. Change is a spiral, and people may move forward and backward, up and down through various stages. Linear progression is rare; only about 5% move through change without setbacks (Prochaska, 1994).

- *Practice mindfulness, compassion, and deep listening to discover what is happening with your clients in the moment.* Are they ready for a plan of action? Or are they unsure why they have been "encouraged" to come to coaching? Are they confident and motivated, with a keen awareness of their larger values and vision for life? Or are they demoralized and doubtful because of past failed attempts? Practicing mindful awareness and using reflective listening will help you recognize the stage or stages your client is in for that behavior. This recognition will guide you as you collaborate on a focus for coaching.
- *Suspend the fixing reflex and the desire to fix.* The effective coach remembers the importance of the working alliance as you talk together and explore choices for a focus. Coaches allow clients to explore and discover where they want to begin the change process. You are not the fixer, the healer, or the changer. Instead, you create an environment where change is possible and supported. This MI-consistent directional orientation occurs in the focusing task.
- *The goal is transformational change.* Changers need support throughout the journey to make and sustain changes. The ultimate end of coaching is for clients to become self-regulated and sustain change over time. Change sometimes involves *doing* something different (transactional). However, professional coaching involves a more encompassing focus on an individual's life and who they are *being*. When people have shifted from deep within, sparked by their intrinsic motivation, and aligned actions with their values, they have had a transformational change that endures. They can apply their learning and insight to new situations throughout their lives. As a coach, keep this larger perspective in view and support your clients to tie goals and action steps back to their broader visions and values, to who they want to be in the future.

CHOOSING A FOCUS IN MI AND COACHING

What should you and your client focus on? Generally, three scenarios present a springboard for moving forward: when the focus is clear, when there are several options to choose from, and when the focus is still unclear.

A Clear Focus

Clients might come with a clear direction in mind: "I want to manage my weight." Or the focus may be implied because of the type of service provided, such as a diabetes management clinic. Or you may uncover a specific direction based on the initial conversations: "You mentioned your difficulty with a fellow worker, and you also want to find ways to be more organized at home. Let's explore which would be most important to you right now."

What happens if you and your client do not initially agree on the focus, or the client lacks clarity on the topic? It is not inconsistent in a client-centered approach for you to offer your own ideas about which direction to go. But the clients' ideas come first and you will emphasize their autonomy in this process. You ask permission to raise the topic, and then the two of you will go exploring.

Use MI-consistent coaching to evoke your clients' intrinsic motivations and possibly open the door for developing discrepancies between current behaviors and values. (Chapter 12 will explore techniques for planting seeds of discrepancy.) In doing so, you remain open-minded and curious in a nonjudgmental way while clients are allowed to enlarge their awareness and perspective. This process is collaborative, and the MI spirit (the coaches' CAPE) sets the tone for doing the work.

Several Options for a Focus

Some clients may have several options to choose from. The question in this case is: Where do you want to start? For example:

> A newly employed night-shift nurse loves her job but worries about being dependent on sleep aids for daytime rest and then stimulants for the night shift. She eats the food in the nurses' lounge to help her stay alert but notices the carbs are causing weight gain. Her doctor told her she was prediabetic. She wishes her spouse would cooperate more to help create a quiet home for daytime sleep. She is concerned about their frequent arguments.

Does the client want to focus on being dependent on sleep aids, or weight gain, or arguing with her spouse?

Or what about a college student who wants to start his career and worries that taking an extra semester to finish undergrad is taking the easy way out? He feels like he will have failed if he does not finish in 4 years, and he stresses about grad school applications, knowing he would have to make new friends and find new roommates if he does not finish in 4 years.

Here, you exercise caution to avoid jumping in with an assumed focus, which may limit your clients' engagement. One method to help guide you in this situation where many issues are on the table is what Miller and Rollnick have called "choosing a path" (2023). We use the term "path finding," as it seems to resonate with clients. (More on choosing a path in the "Path-Finding Tool" section, below.)

When the Focus Is Unclear

"There are so many things I need help with, and I'm confused." Clients may come with a gunnysack full of seemingly unrelated issues. Your job is to orient the session by reviewing these options and then working together to prioritize the collection. The broad focus becomes increasingly narrower.

A more directional (not directive) guiding style can facilitate choosing a focus. Just listening and following along is not enough. Infuse your guidance with your and your client's respective expertise and knowledge; you are equal partners. As a coach, you gently align (guide) the pieces, moving closer and closer to what might resemble an array of reasonable paths to take. Several paths become more apparent with your guidance, but collaboration remains a priority. This task of focusing is rich with OARS and robust listening while you sensitively guide your client toward clarity.

The end target, the longer-range goals, or the broader life vision define the general direction. Align the long- and short-range goals and action steps toward this direction. The end destination is kept in sight along this trajectory and becomes the north star for which path or paths to take. The distinctions made here may not always be this clear in your practice, but this discussion provides a general framework for the focusing task.

MI METHODS AND TOOLS FOR EXPLORING FOCUS

Longer-Term Goals, Values, and Vision

Miller and Rollnick (2023) suggested several methods for exploring focus, such as identifying clients' longer-term goals, which provide context for motivation and the work to come. In MI and coaching, these goals are linked to what people value and what is important to them. Those larger life goals are a source of motivation for change, pulling clients forward. Juxtaposing longer-term goals with clients' everyday experience can also unearth discrepancies that exert powerful force on behaviors.

You cannot install motivation. But spending time exploring what is most important to your clients—their values, purpose, and the meaning in their lives, and what they aspire to—is time well spent. These provide the keys to finding out what motivates them.

Initial Conversation

During an initial conversation, good reflective listening can provide more insight into a client than a written, presession intake assessment does. Although the written form provides basic information, if it is too data-heavy it might imply that clients will assume a passive role while you sort the information and make a plan. Clients' early impressions of how the coaching relationship will function will help build the working alliance that is vital to successful outcomes.

This initial conversation can be one where you invite clients to explore and articulate their values and broader life goals or vision. Use the MI spirit (coaches' CAPE) to infuse the conversation and maintain that mindset as you proceed. Open-ended questions can be used to explore answers to questions such as the following.

"What do you stand for?"
"What is important to you?"
"What guides your life?"
"What are the most important rules you live by?"

Thoughtful reflections and open questions can help broaden clients' ideas about how these values might show up in their everyday lives.

"What are some ways [value] shows up in your life?"
"How has [value] helped determine your life choices?"
"In what ways do you live your life following [value]?"

Personal Values Card Sort

The Personal Values Card Sort activity is a structured way to explore clients' values. In this activity, a coach provides a client with a list of cards, each of which names a value with a short definition of that value. The client sorts the cards into five levels of importance, ranging from not important to most important. The same reflections and questions suggested above can help deepen a client's perspective about their own values, which sharpens the focus for the upcoming work. (See the Personal Values Card Sort Activity available at *www.guilford.com/companion-site/Motivational-Interviewing-Fourth-Edition/9781462552795*.)

COACHING METHODS FOR EXPLORING FOCUS

Taking a cue from MI, you first zoom out to capture a broader view of clients' aspirations, dreams, life purpose, and vision for their lives. Then, you use MI methods to help narrow down a focus for the overall coaching engagement and individual sessions. The broader perspective becomes a positive force that places long- and short-term goals in context. (See more details in Chapter 6.)

Initial Visit

Like in MI, you as a coach might begin this exploration process on the first visit, either by phone or in person; this is often called a "discovery session"

(Kimsey-House et al., 2018). You can ask questions to tease out a person's broader perspective: "Imagine that you are living your best life. In this life, what qualities do you possess? What relationships do you have? How do you picture yourself?"

You may begin to plant the seeds of the working alliance: "What is the best way for me to coach you?" Or you might start talking about values: "What would you say are values you live by?" You could ask about possible areas of focus: "Name three to five areas you might choose as your main focus during the coaching relationship."

Path-Finding Tool

As discussed above, when there are several options on the table for focusing on in your sessions, you, as coach, will resist the urge to decide which one takes priority. Instead, foster a working alliance by involving the client and building engagement. A possible sequence for that engagement is to list the options, evaluate the choices, and then agree on a focus. Your task is to walk collaboratively alongside an autonomous client.

The path-finding tool is a method for zooming out to consider the way forward with a specific focus. Once all the options are listed in the tool, the two of you begin to zero in on what the client feels would be the best initial focus. Below is a sequence Miller and Rollnick (2023) have suggested for using the tool to choose the route for the journey ahead.

First, state that you and your client will step back and survey the options to get clear on a direction. Ask permission to explore the possibilities with an open-ended and invitational tone.

> "You mentioned on our initial visit that you want to eat fewer carbs and lose weight, and your doctor said you have prediabetes. Other things seem to be important to you also right now. You're concerned about taking sleeping aids, you need a quiet environment for sleeping at home during the daytime, and you and your spouse are arguing. Where do you think we should start?"

Next, invite the client to verbally explore the options. You can offer your ideas, with permission, perhaps based on observations made during the initial conversation. The use of visual aids such as a simple checklist, a brainstorm-mapping activity, or a graphic like the path-finding tool with shapes to write in are some ways to organize the ideas. Referring back to visual aids in future sessions can serve as an anchor for checking in and asking about changes or modifications to the focus. These visual anchors can become landmarks to help stay the course. (See Figure 5.2 for a sample of this activity. Handout 5.1 is a blank version, available at *www.guilford.com/lanier-materials*.)

Directions: Use this form to help you narrow down one topic from among several of your ideas for a single session. It can also be used to help you choose a few broader areas to focus on for your entire coaching arrangement.

Write one topic in each of the hexagons provided. (Use a few or all of the hexagons.) Then, you might want to prioritize your topics numerically, as shown below. (Use the small boxes.) Afterward, you will have a conversation with your coach to help clarify your chosen topic for exploration and work.

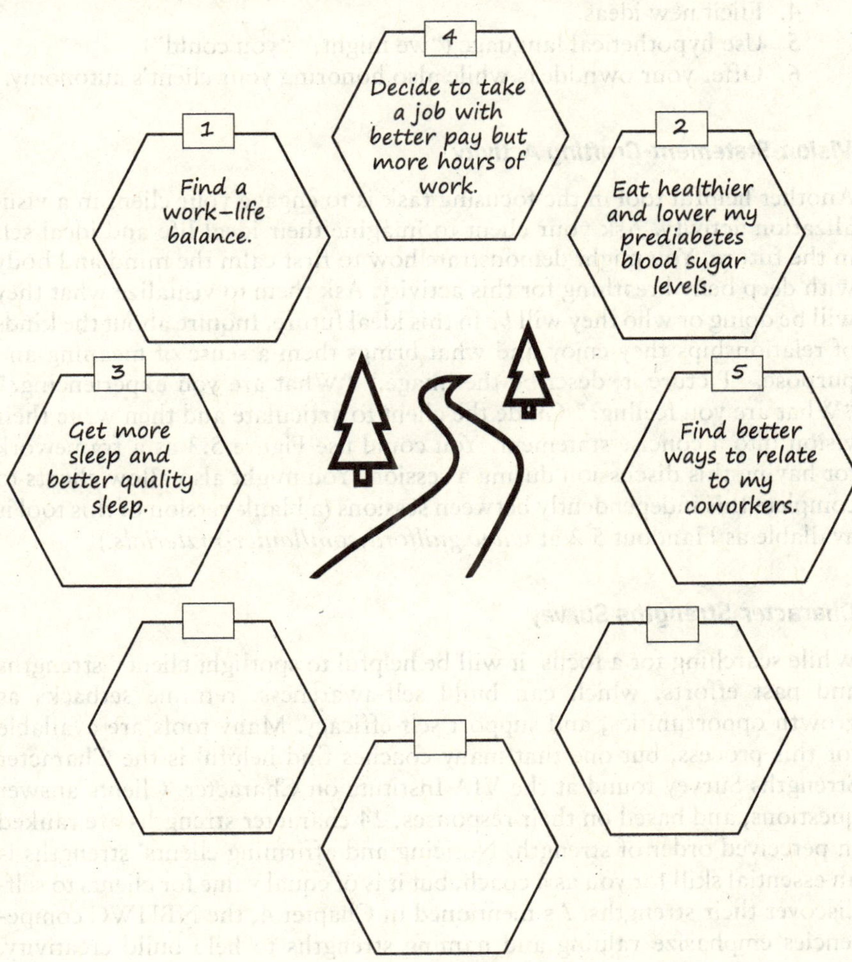

FIGURE 5.2. A partially completed path-finding tool.

Here's a suggested list of guidelines for using the path-finding tool during the focusing task (Miller & Rollnick, 2023):

1. Invite, wait, give space.
2. Affirm, support.
3. Highlight strengths and emphasize autonomy.
4. Elicit new ideas.
5. Use hypothetical language ("we might," "you could").
6. Offer your own ideas while also honoring your client's autonomy.

Vision-Statement-Crafting Activity

Another helpful tool in the focusing task is to engage your client in a visualization activity. Ask your client to imagine their ideal life and ideal self in the future. You might demonstrate how to first calm the mind and body with deep belly breathing for this activity. Ask them to visualize what they will be doing or who they will *be* in this ideal future. Inquire about the kinds of relationships they enjoy and what brings them a sense of meaning and purpose. "Picture it, describe the image." "What are you experiencing?" "What are you feeling?" Guide the client to articulate and then write their vision into a concise statement. You could use Figure 5.3 as a framework for having this discussion during a session. You might also allow clients to complete this independently between sessions (a blank version of this tool is available as Handout 5.2 at *www.guilford.com/lanier-materials.*)

Character Strengths Survey

While searching for a focus, it will be helpful to spotlight clients' strengths and past efforts, which can build self-awareness, reframe setbacks as growth opportunities, and support self-efficacy. Many tools are available for this process, but one that many coaches find helpful is the Character Strengths Survey found at the VIA Institute on Character. Clients answer questions, and based on their responses, 24 character strengths are ranked in perceived order of strength. Noticing and affirming clients' strengths is an essential skill for you as a coach, but it is of equal value for clients to self-discover their strengths. As mentioned in Chapter 4, the NBHWC competencies emphasize valuing and naming strengths to help build creativity, open-mindedness, strategic thinking, resilience, and connection.

Offer reflections that tie clients' values and strengths back to potential goals or desired outcomes. Open-ended questions can help clients connect strengths to their overall vision and purpose or sense of meaning in life. "What strengths could you use to achieve your vision?" "What strengths were you using when you achieved a goal that you value?" (Readers can

Directions:

- This form can be started in a coaching session and completed either during that session or before the next session. You will invite the client to reflect on the Explore and Dream boxes and ask them to write responses in the corresponding boxes on the right.
- Once the client has written several responses in Boxes 2 and 3, ask them to create a summary statement that encapsulates the vision they created for their best self in their ideal future. (A sample vision statement is provided below.)

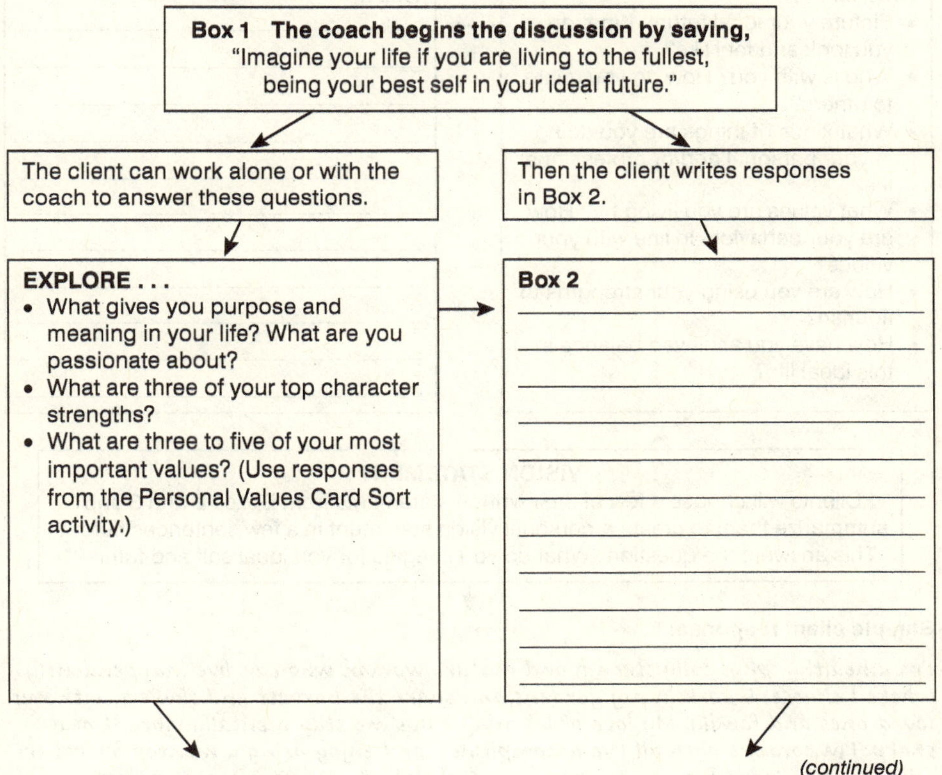

Box 1 The coach begins the discussion by saying,
"Imagine your life if you are living to the fullest, being your best self in your ideal future."

The client can work alone or with the coach to answer these questions.

Then the client writes responses in Box 2.

EXPLORE . . .

- What gives you purpose and meaning in your life? What are you passionate about?
- What are three of your top character strengths?
- What are three to five of your most important values? (Use responses from the Personal Values Card Sort activity.)

Box 2

(continued)

FIGURE 5.3. Designing a personal vision statement.

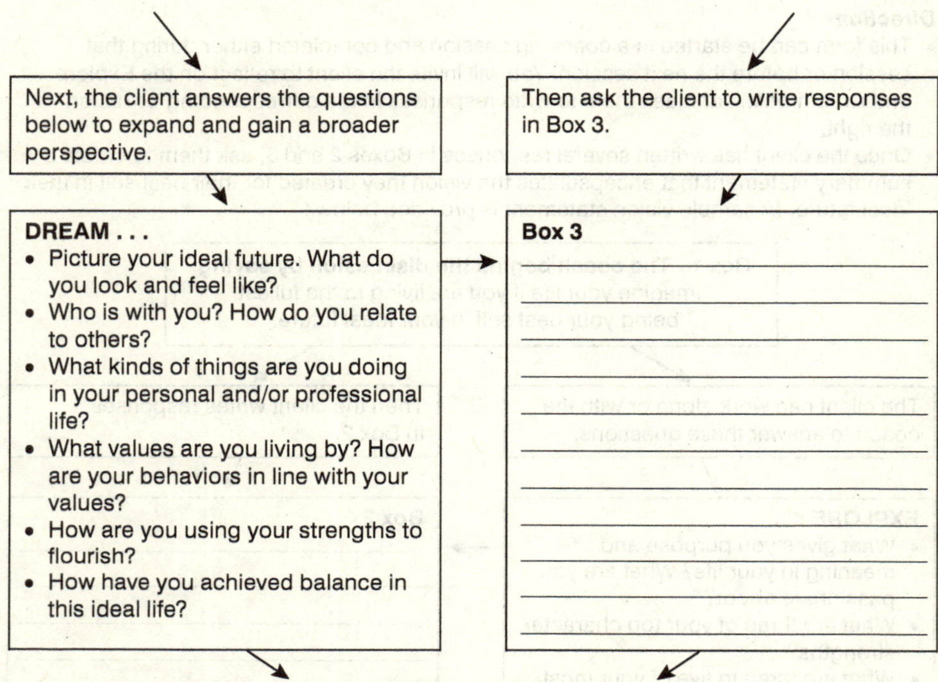

Next, the client answers the questions below to expand and gain a broader perspective.
Then ask the client to write responses in Box 3.
DREAM . . .
• Picture your ideal future. What do you look and feel like?
• Who is with you? How do you relate to others?
• What kinds of things are you doing in your personal and/or professional life?
• What values are you living by? How are your behaviors in line with your values?
• How are you using your strengths to flourish?
• How have you achieved balance in this ideal life?
Box 3
VISION STATEMENT
Clients will choose a few of their written statements from Boxes 2 and 3 and summarize them to create a personal vision statement in a few sentences below. This answers the question "What do you imagine for you ideal self and future?"

Sample client response:

I'm a healthy, physically strong, and mature woman who can live independently where I choose. I work in my gardens and share the harvest and flowers with my loved ones and family. My love of learning helps me stay mentally vibrant and sharp. I'm content with all I've accomplished and enjoy being a mentor for others who want to learn from my experience and skills. I stay connected with my family and a group of people who also like to learn, enjoy nature and keep learning and growing.

FIGURE 5.3. *(continued)*

find a link to the free online VIA Character Strengths Survey at *www.guilford.com/lanier-materials.*)

Wheel of Life Tool

Homeostasis is a state of equilibrium in the physical and psychological realms. Our bodies regulate temperature and other functions to maintain physiological balance in the body. Psychological homeostasis is the human tendency to desire a state of emotional balance, stability, and equilibrium so that one functions with congruence at an optimal level (Cummins, 2013). Your clients most likely seek coaching due to a perceived imbalance in one or more areas of their lives.

The Wheel of Life is an effective tool that is often used in discovery sessions to help clients view a snapshot of how balanced and fulfilled they feel in their lives. The Wheel of Life has the potential to point clients in the direction of finding which area of focus is most important to them.

A circle is divided into eight or nine pie-shaped pieces, which you may choose to personalize with categories fit to a client's needs. The commonly used categories are career, physical environment, fun and recreation, significant other/romance, personal growth and development, friendships, family, health and well-being, and finances.

Ask clients to rank their current level of satisfaction in each area on a scale of 1 to 10 (with 10 being fully satisfied). After clients connect the lines from each category to create an inner "circle," the coach then asks, "How well does your wheel roll?" We find this tool often elicits an audible "Wow!" from clients, and they share more about the areas of balance and imbalance. They find clarity and can more easily answer the question, "What area would you like to focus on?"

The Wheel of Life can also be used at a final session as a subjective measurement of client progress and growth. The client will most likely have forgotten the responses from the first session. The coach can ask, "Do you mind if we go through the Wheel of Life again?" Inquiring about the client's current level of fulfillment for each area, the client or the coach marks their responses on their original Wheel of Life with a different color pen. Once the second wheel is drawn, compare the two wheels, showing the difference between the first session and the final session. Clients often are delighted with the progress they have made. (See Figure 5.4. A blank version of this tool can be found in Handout 5.3 at *www.guilford.com/lanier-materials.*)

Finalizing the Focus

Checking in to make sure you have covered all possible options can be prompted with a few questions: "Does this include all your concerns?" "Would there be any other areas we should consider?" "How are you

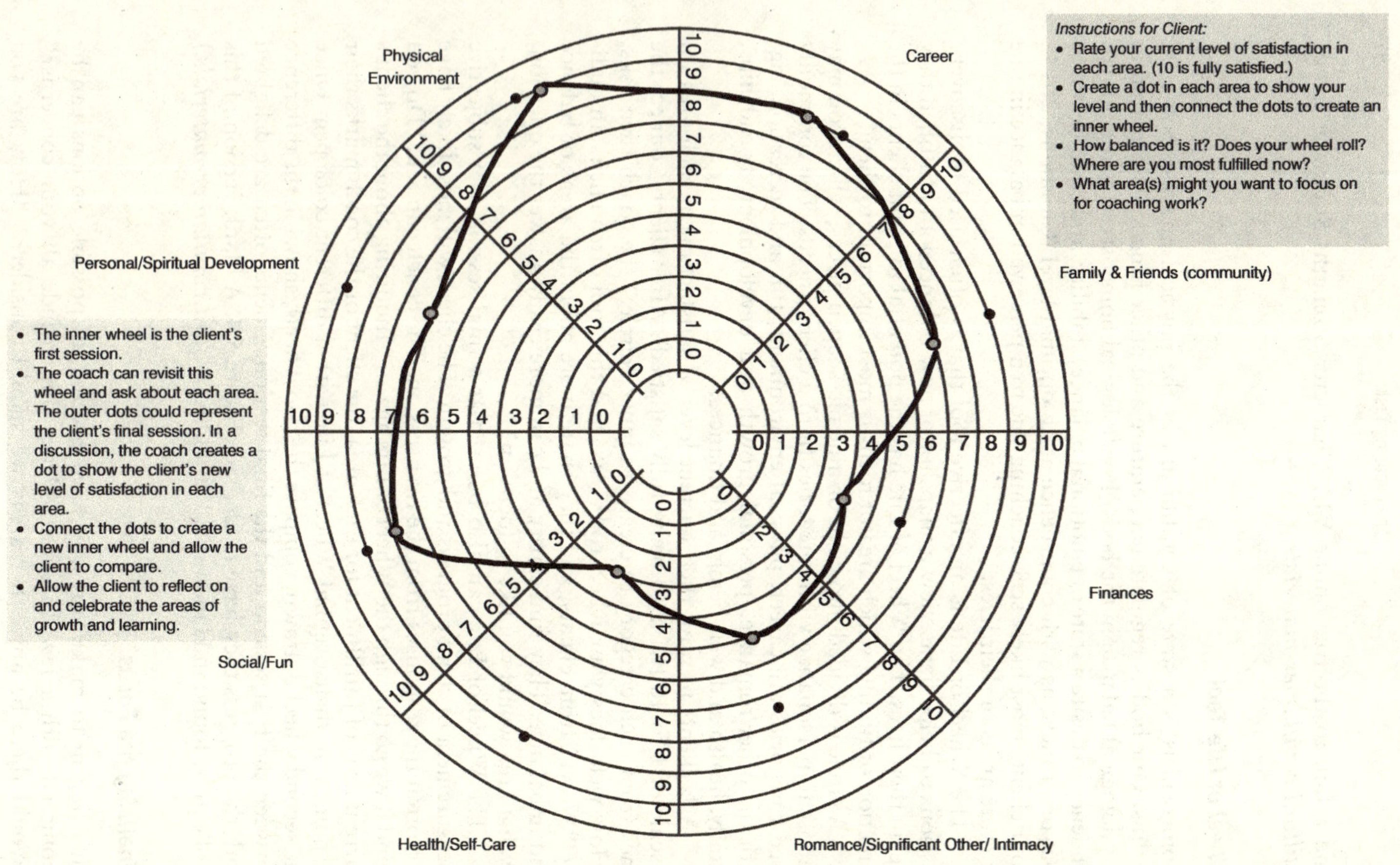

Instructions for Client:
• Rate your current level of satisfaction in each area. (10 is fully satisfied.)
• Create a dot in each area to show your level and then connect the dots to create an inner wheel.
• How balanced is it? Does your wheel roll? Where are you most fulfilled now?
• What area(s) might you want to focus on for coaching work?
Career
Family & Friends (community)
Finances
Romance/Significant Other/ Intimacy
Health/Self-Care
Social/Fun
Personal/Spiritual Development
Physical Environment
• The inner wheel is the client's first session.
• The coach can revisit this wheel and ask about each area. The outer dots could represent the client's final session. In a discussion, the coach creates a dot to show the client's new level of satisfaction in each area.
• Connect the dots to create a new inner wheel and allow the client to compare.
• Allow the client to reflect on and celebrate the areas of growth and learning.

FIGURE 5.4. A partially completed Wheel of Life tool.

feeling about this direction?" Finally, when you land on a target and agree on the direction, use the MI skill of summarizing to assist clients to confirm and clarify the focus. Now that the primary area of concern is identified, this becomes the starting point for the journey.

Take It Further

Directions: Work with your learning community to read and respond to questions 1–4 below. Locate Handout 5.4 online at *www.guilford.com/lanier-materials*, and use it to answer question 4c.

1. Define the major distinctions between the roles of coaches and the roles of counselors, therapists, and mentors.
2. Within your group, discuss the purpose of the focusing task. Then, define and list the main jobs for you, the coach, in the focusing task. What is most important to consider?
3. Consider this client (below), who chose financial goals for the topic to work on in this session. How might you "focus and refocus" the conversation? Remember to emphasize autonomy.

   "We had to deal with the death of our dog this week. It was so upsetting that it made me want to reset everything in the house. I think I'd like to plan for organizing my bedroom closet. I love shoes, and I have a lot! And then, I want to decide how I'm going to organize the pantry for the holidays. I've been avoiding that."
4. Download Handout 5.4, Vision, Goals, and Action Steps. The term "positive emotional attractors" (Boyatzis et al., 2019) refers to those positive things that inspire people to move forward. (See Vision bubble in the handout.)
   a. Ideally, when might you prefer to ask your clients about their vision of their ideal self and future? Discuss this with your group.
   b. Long- and short-term goals are often completed through a series of action steps. Consider how focusing on action steps first might jeopardize sustainable change.
   c. MI-consistent coaching emphasizes connecting your clients' goals with a larger vision. Use the graphic on Handout 5.4 as a guide and describe the "hierarchy of goals" mentioned earlier in this chapter.

Chapter 6

Evoking Motivation

Evoking is the third of the four tasks of MI practice. In the engaging task, you connected with your clients to build a working alliance (Chapter 4). Reflective listening helped you mirror back what they said while communicating that you sought to understand their perspective. Using OARS (open questions, affirmation, reflections, and summaries) demonstrated empathy and invited clients to explore more of their dilemmas. Your authentic affirmations kept the focus on your clients' positive qualities, strengths, and efforts. You called upon effective positive psychology models and emphasized what is right with your client versus what is wrong. You built the working alliance in an atmosphere where the MI spirit (the coaches' CAPE) set the tone for the conversations. Clients felt safe exploring their perspectives within this collaborative, nonjudgmental, confidential, and compassionate relationship.

In the focusing task (Chapter 5), you continued using OARS to invite and guide the client on a journey of collaboratively finding a direction for the sessions. You resisted the fixing reflex and instead honored each client's autonomy to choose their focus and related goals. You agreed on a destination toward which the work would be focused. Your clients spent time exploring their values and a larger vision for their ideal selves and futures. In focusing, you pointed the way to each client's destination, guiding them on the journey of self-discovery and insight for the strategic path ahead.

This third task, evoking, is what differentiates MI from other approaches. A noticeable shift occurs when you use OARS in a directional way. Many other methods use the skills we discussed in engaging and focusing, but MI practice is unique because of the evoking task. The helper becomes explicitly directional (but not directive) to evoke motivation. By this, we mean that you will use the same OARS skills in a slightly different way and for another reason.

Instead of a purely client-focused, following style, MI implants a goal-oriented method that gives special consideration to the client's language of change for the purpose of their eventual change. This goal-oriented approach fits squarely into the context of coaching, as expressed by coach Meg Jordan: "Coaching is a supportive alliance that allows the client to expand . . . and experiment with life-changing behaviors that lead to the fulfillment of client goals" (2022). Your support provides the guardrails for this work, and the MI skill of evoking becomes the *way* you help clients find and strengthen their own motivations for reaching their goals. The MI skill of evoking fits hand-in-glove with the coaching skills of cultivating intrinsic motivation (NBHWC) and facilitating client growth (ICF).

MI practice elicits, explores, and strengthens what is already there: the clients' own motivations for change. Evoking clients' talk about change and inviting more of it raises the likelihood that clients will make a change (Moyers et al., 2009). Helpers do not insert motivation; evoking implies that what is necessary for change already exists within a person. As an MI-consistent coach, your task is to call it forth, stoke the flame, ignite the embers, or whatever metaphor helps you conceptualize this process. What is needed within your clients' often-subdued awareness is to awaken and bring their internal motivation to life.

We are sure that as a coach, you can easily spot the parallels between the evoking task of MI and coaching. You are a guide who does more than merely listen to and empathize with clients; you provide structure while supporting them to move toward their goals. MI-consistent coaching is *how* you evoke clients' motivation—first to consider, then to plan (see Chapter 13, on planning), and finally to make a change. In the evoking task, you actively influence the course of the conversation.

Recall the coaches' paradoxes in Chapter 1, which asked, "How can I help someone if I shouldn't tell them what to do?" "If this is a client-led approach, what role do I play in helping them move toward change?" The answers lie in understanding the skill of evoking. Those questions uncover seeming inconsistencies, but our discussion of the evoking skill can bring clarity to your role of facilitating client growth and cultivating intrinsic motivation. The evoking skills address *how* you can facilitate the process.

As discussed, MI practice helps clients express their motivations for change (their why), explore their discrepancies, resolve their ambivalence, and strengthen their own arguments and subsequent actions for change. To be motivated to change and simultaneously motivated to stay the same is ambivalence, which is a natural step on the path toward change.

AMBIVALENCE

Motivation exists in two realms: wanting to stay the same while simultaneously wanting to move out of that sameness toward a change. Ambivalence is the normal expression of this dichotomy, arguing for and against change. Once clients voice these internal arguments in a coaching session, you recognize them for what they are: clients' arguments about whether to change and whether the change is considered possible and worth the effort. Learning the skill of evoking will help you become attentive to the language and degree of ambivalence and provide ways to respond to increase the likelihood of change.

What about clients who do not seem to be ambivalent? Some clients who are somewhat satisfied with a particular behavior may signal that they have little to no intention (yet) to change; they seem to have no language about change to evoke, at least for that behavior. For example, a doctor prescribes dietary changes to his patient and suggests the patient visit a coach for support. But when the patient becomes a coaching client, they verbalize concern around stress management instead. When you inquire about this, you might hear, "I think my diet is healthy right now, so I'd prefer to work on stress."

The client's language reflects satisfaction with the status quo (about dietary changes), and "change talk" is almost absent. This person is in the precontemplation stage of change (see the discussion of "The Stages of Change" in Chapter 5) and is possibly unaware that a problem exists, having little or no ambivalence about the behavior. In this case, Miller and Rollnick suggest an approach they call "planting seeds," which helps you explore clients' ambivalence (2023). We will revisit and expand on this approach in Chapter 12.

As people move out of the precontemplation stage into contemplation, you can hear the inner debate, which bubbles to the surface as they express it in their language. However, use caution in labeling them as "ambivalent," as if they have a pathology. Ambivalence is a normal step toward change. Your best tactic is to resist judgment while inviting this ambivalence to surface within the safe environment you created in the coaching relationship.

Human experience affirms the disquieting impact of this internal dialogue, where two sides each make their case. Internal arguments for the pros or cons sides of change can stir a great deal of discomfort. A first-century author poured out his lament about his internal ambivalence: "For I do not understand my own actions. I do not do what I want, but I do the very thing I hate" (ESV Study Bible, 2016). Your role is to invite these internal arguments to be voiced out loud by your clients so that each side of their arguments get a "day in court."

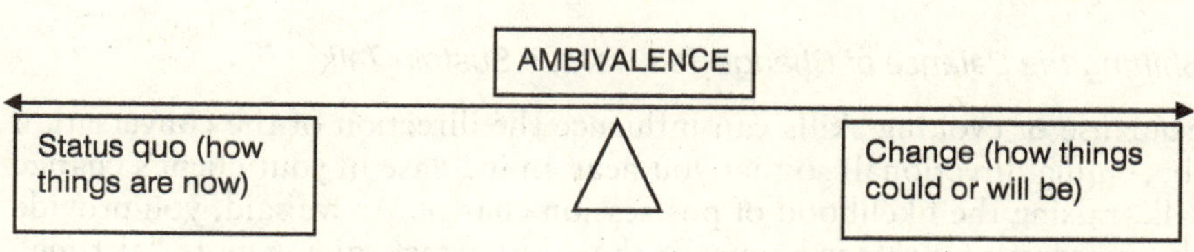

FIGURE 6.1. Ambivalence.

As clients voice these debates, you will often hear the conjunction *but* inserted between pro and con statements, which indicates ambivalence about a behavior change.

> "I have to stop eating fast food, *but we're all going to die of something; this is my thing.*"
>
> "I can make some small changes to get going, *but it won't make a difference.*"
>
> "Yes, doing something might help, *but I've tried everything, and nothing works.*"
>
> "I need to stop these negative thoughts, *but I'm just a negative person; it's who I am.*"

Attempts to escape discomfort muffle this internal chatter. But when the whispered debate is hushed, clients can perpetuate the status quo and remain stuck in this state of contemplation. Some (or many) of your clients come to the coaching relationship in this stage of change, and you can use your sense of compassion to connect with and show empathy for them. Ambivalence is a common human experience (Figure 6.1).

The Coach's Role in Ambivalence

Listening well is a foundational skill for the practice of MI and indeed for the service of coaching, but listening is not where the evoking task ends. People experiencing ambivalence need the opportunity to express their change talk, and it is a coach's privilege to invite and elicit more of it. Research confirms that clients are more likely to change when their voiced arguments for change outweigh their arguments to stay the same (Magill et al., 2018).

In addition to empathy, the skill of evoking exerts the most significant influence on clients' movement toward change, helping them resolve their ambivalence and move past the contemplation stage toward planning. A coach's use of evoking can increase the amount and strength of clients' pro-change arguments (change talk) while decreasing the arguments to stay the same (sustain talk).

Shifting the Balance of Change Talk versus Sustain Talk

Your use of evoking skills can influence the direction of the conversation (becoming directional) so that you hear an increase in your client's change talk, raising the likelihood of postsession change. As we said, you provide the guardrails for this to happen in the evoking task, giving more "airtime" to the person's own arguments for change (Moyers & Martin, 2006; Moyers et al., 2009).

One caveat is that although more change talk increases the likelihood of change, the adverse is also true; the more clients verbalize their sustain talk, the more likely they will sustain their behavior (Magill et al., 2019; Apodaca et al., 2014). So, what you pay attention to and reflect on matters.

The balance of client change talk to sustain talk is one indicator of readiness to change, and your goal is to increase this ratio to more change talk than sustain talk. The key takeaway for your work as a coach is that what you say can influence and tilt this balance of change talk and sustain talk in either direction (Gaume et al., 2010).

Glynn and Moyers (2010) devised a study to test the hypothesis that clinicians can influence change talk. If clinicians intentionally evoked change talk, would clients' change talk increase in frequency? If clinicians

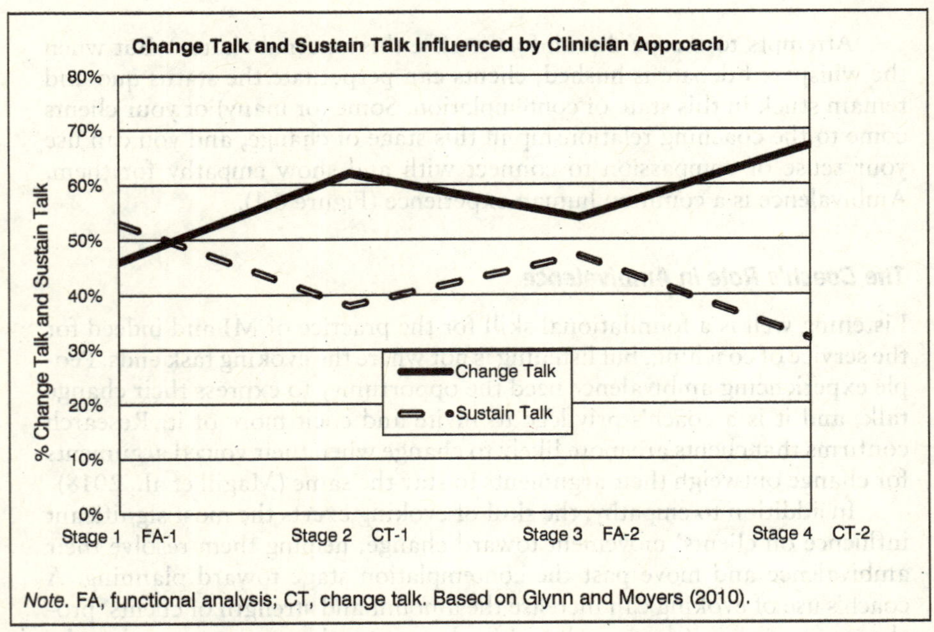

Note. FA, functional analysis; CT, change talk. Based on Glynn and Moyers (2010).

FIGURE 6.2. Change talk and sustain talk influenced by clinician approach. *Note.* FA, functional analysis; CT, change talk. Based on Glynn and Moyers (2010).

used other strategies, would change talk decrease? The study defined two types of conditions: one where clinicians use questions designed to evoke change talk (CT) and the other where clinicians used fact-gathering questions to determine triggering causes and consequences of the problem behavior (functional analysis [FA]). The study observed the frequency of client change talk as counselors used the two strategies during four stages.

Figure 6.2 depicts the relative rise and fall in change talk as a result of using either FA or CT. The data support the theory that when clinicians intentionally evoked and strengthened change talk (CT), the clients' change talk increased. When clinicians used the other method (FA), the change talk decreased.

TWO IMPORTANT QUESTIONS: "WHY?" AND "HOW TO CHANGE?"

After the *what* of change is established in the focusing task, changers are concerned with two other questions: "*Why* is this change important to me?" and "*How* would I do it?" You may hear the perceived importance of a potential change in these types of statements.

"It's not life or death, but I sure would feel better if I did this."
"I need to do something. This inflammation is too hard on my joints."
"If I want to stay employed, I have to improve my productivity."

Change is often challenging, so before people put forth the effort, they usually have good reasons to do it, with plenty of "want to" mixed in and some measure of urgency about it. Addressing the second question, the *how* of change typically follows the *why*. Practically speaking, this implies that after evoking clients' motivation to change, you proceed to evoking a plan for change (discussed in Chapter 13).

But what about those clients who are acutely aware of the high importance of a particular change and yet remain stuck because they cannot imagine where to start or have faced repeated failed attempts? They have very low confidence despite the perceived importance. The clients' confidence in their ability to change will impact their efforts, since confidence is a necessary component of self-determination (Ryan & Deci, 2008). In this case, the first order of business is to evoke confidence (discussed in Chapter 10).

THE SOUND OF CHANGE TALK

You can hear someone's intention to change in the nuances of language, and based on what you hear, you sense where they are on the journey toward an action. When people consider change, you hear change talk in varying degrees, and they may be somewhere between a soft consideration on one end and taking steps toward action on the other. Notice the strength of the intentions in these statements and try to determine the level of change talk.

"Don't ask me; I'm not skilled at installing appliances."
"I'm not interested in learning that skill."
"That will take a lot of work; I'll think about it."
"I don't see a problem with doing that."
"I could probably figure out how to install it."
"Maybe I can figure that out."
"I might come by and look at it. I am almost positive I can do it."
"I will come by next week and bring my tools."

Preparatory Change Talk

MI has a helpful way of categorizing seven types of change talk into two broad categories: preparatory change talk and mobilizing change talk. Preparatory change talk describes language that demonstrates a consideration of change. The car engine is on with the gear in neutral, and the motor is revving up and preparing to move. You begin chugging up the hill of change, which takes some concerted effort.

Miller and Rollnick (2023) used the acronym DARN to help us recognize these statements as expressions of desire, ability, reason, and need for change. Clients' language gives clues about their readiness to change, revealing the perceived level of importance of the change, their reasons for change, and their sense of confidence that they can make the change happen. Here are some examples of preparatory change talk.

Desire

Some words used to depict desire are *want, like, wish,* and *love.* In these, you hear some desire toward action.

"I *want* to stop drinking wine every night."
"I would *like* to get back to swimming every day."
"I *wish* I could get this weight off and keep it off."
"I would *love* to feel confident about my work."

Ability

These statements uncover people's level of confidence in acting toward change. Words that indicate ability are *can, could, able, possible,* and *try.*

"I *can* get a journal and start recording my thoughts."
"I *could* pack my swim bag the night before."
"I'm *able* to organize my time better."
"It's *possible* to shut down technology earlier in the evening."
"I'll *try* to eliminate gluten and dairy next week." (Notice that the *try* statement hints at some doubt about the ability to do it.)

Reasons

This kind of preparatory change talk articulates the reasons someone may do something, and you often hear it expressed as if–then statements. Reasons make a case for the pros of change or the cons of not changing.

"If I keep my blood sugar level, then I might have more focus at work."
"My wife can't do the work alone, so my fitness level could support her."
"If I used meditation, I would hopefully be calmer during stressful days."
"The right kind of support would keep me encouraged to keep going."

Need

Need statements express the importance or urgency of a change. (When a need statement includes a *why* it is a reason.)

"I have to get this house organized."
"I need to prioritize sleep."
"I've got to have a sit-down meeting with my team."
"I absolutely need to lower my stress."

Mobilizing Change Talk

"Mobilizing" implies people are starting to show an inclination, a movement toward a certain change. As the car reaches the hilltop after working on the preparatory change talk, acceleration increases, and momentum drives the path toward change. People's language indicates they are gaining traction on the journey from the earlier preparatory change talk. The acronym CATs helps you remember the three additional types of change talk you hear as people consider action: commitment, activation, and taking steps.

Note: A logical progression of mobilizing change talk could be viewed as commitment talk in order of strength. In this case, we would order them from activation (leaning toward), commitment (considering how), and then taking steps (doing something), or ACTs. But we find the acronym DARN

CATs a bit easier to remember. Cat lovers can testify to the difficulty of calling those DARN CATs!

Commitment

A strong form of mobilizing change talk is commitment language that holds a level of assurance that things will happen. Clients declare something will happen, and these statements of intent can range from soft promises to solid, more robust levels of commitment.

"I *will* do it."
"I *promise* I'm going to learn this habit."
"I *guarantee* I'm starting this tomorrow."
"I *swear* I'm going to make this happen."

Activation

Activation statements indicate the person's inclination and openness toward change, though they have not yet made a firm decision or commitment. It's a slight leaning, but it's leaning nonetheless and an encouraging sign that change is considered. These are not the strong types of declarations one hears in a contract or a vow such as, "I promise to be faithful to you." Although activation statements are milder statements, the good news is that all change talk matters and predicts change; it is not necessary to hear commitment.

"I *could* probably do it."
"I would *consider* it."
"I'm *thinking* about doing it."

Taking Steps

This type of language signals that the person has taken some action toward change, however small.

"I downloaded an app for nighttime meditation."
"I called three schools and asked about their massage therapy program."
"I cleaned out the pantry and got rid of all the junk."

Increased change talk during a session may be your signal that the client is resolving ambivalence and ready for preparation to plan. You will make a judgment call about whether there is enough change talk and if you perceive their readiness to shift. If you are dubious, you can always check your guess and ask. (More about this in Chapter 13.)

COACH: You said you need to follow your doctor's cardiometabolic diet, and you downloaded the plan, and you wanted help sticking to the plan. Are you ready to start taking steps?

CLIENT: Yeah, but as I'm talking, I think the most urgent problem is my upcoming shoulder surgery. I can't concentrate on the diet now with all that stress.

THE SOUND OF SUSTAIN TALK

In ambivalence, the counterpoint to change talk is arguments for staying the same, or what MI calls sustain talk, which is categorized using the same DARN CATs labels. Both change talk and sustain talk refer to the arguments one makes regarding a specific change. Desire, ability, reason, and need statements are voiced in favor of staying the same (sustain talk) or making a change (change talk). The same is true for commitment statements.

	Change Talk	*Sustain Talk*
Desire:	"I *want* to stress less."	"I really *thrive* in chaos."
Ability:	"I *can* learn some strategies."	"I *can't* imagine sitting still for meditation."
Reasons:	"If I relaxed, my health could improve."	"If I relax, I stress over what didn't get done."
Need:	"I need to slow down and relax."	"I need the stimulation of activity."
Activation:	"I'm willing to learn meditation."	"I'm planning to just stick to my usual."
Commitment:	"I'll learn meditation to destress."	"I've decided to forgo meditation."
Taking steps:	"I downloaded the sleep app today."	"I scrolled social media to relax before bed."

In reality, change talk and sustain talk are often intermingled and presented as one sentence. Expressions of both pros and cons reveal the conflicting motives.

"I *want* a more peaceful life, but I just *can't* relax."
"I *want* to quit my dependence on chocolate, but I always *crave it*."

THE MI HILL

The flow of an MI conversation described earlier might resemble a hill that shows the likely progression of change talk (see Figure 6.3). First, on the upward slope, you see the DARN statements indicating preparatory change talk or preparation to change. As we said, this preparatory change talk is much like moving uphill, which requires more concentration and energy and may be a slower ascent. Next, you can envision the CATs statements on the mobilizing down slope indicating more intentional movement toward change. As the analogy suggests, going downhill has the benefit of momentum and gravity, and the pace is faster.

Note: Take caution that you honor clients' pace and avoid going too fast in this phase, inadvertently rushing the development of a goal before they are ready. (We discuss this further in Chapter 13.)

When you use MI evoking skills in a session with ambivalent clients, the conversation follows a general progression, indicating movement from less ready to more ready to act. But remember, any change talk is a move in the right direction and is important.

Notice in Figure 6.3 how the flow of change talk corresponds to the stages of change. Change talk is typically absent if a client is in the precontemplation stage regarding a specific behavior. As people progress toward the contemplation and planning stages, one expects to hear more talk about change and then considerations for how to make the change.

As you become more attuned to the amount of change talk versus sustain talk, you will use that awareness to guide your coaching sessions. This awareness enables you, in each moment, to get a feel for which way the scale is tilting. If the distribution is balanced, 50% change talk and 50% sustain talk, you probably intuit that change is not likely to happen (ambivalence).

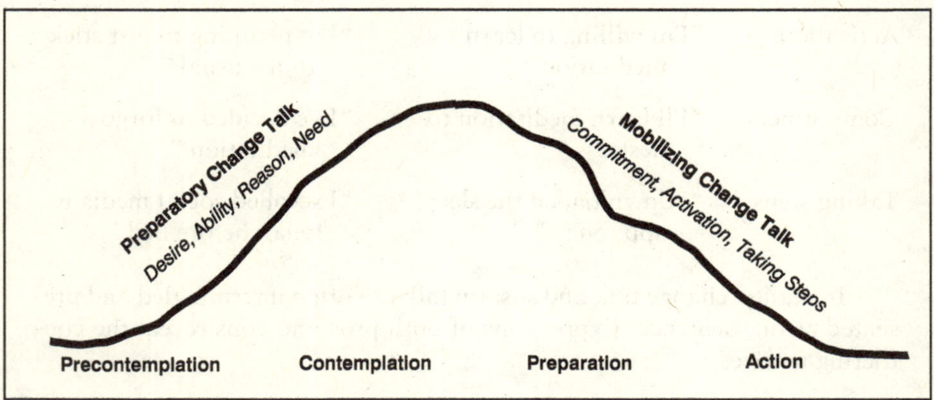

FIGURE 6.3. MI hill.

But if you hear the ratio shift to an increase in change talk and movement toward commitment talk, this indicates that change is more likely.

The Balance of Change Talk to Sustain Talk

The evidence confirms what most people already know; the more you hear someone talking about change, the higher the likelihood they will change. A significant reality to highlight from the research is that sustain talk tends to be a better (inverse) predictor of no change. You may see this in your own practice: The more sustain talk you hear, the more likely it is that your client does not change.

Several studies have demonstrated that an increased ratio of change talk to sustain talk predicts the likelihood of change (Magill et al., 2018; Moyers et al., 2009). Analyses of in-session MI-consistent behaviors showed that client change talk was a predictor of change. Equally significant was the finding that increased client sustain talk was a predictor of staying the same, not changing. It is worth repeating: Listening carefully to what your clients are saying helps you sense which way the balance is tilting and allows you to respond in a way to increase the change talk. Figure 6.4 depicts combined research that tracks clients' change talk progression during sessions. Based on the MI premise that increased change talk predicts after-session change, can you determine which client will most probably change? Which client will likely remain the same?

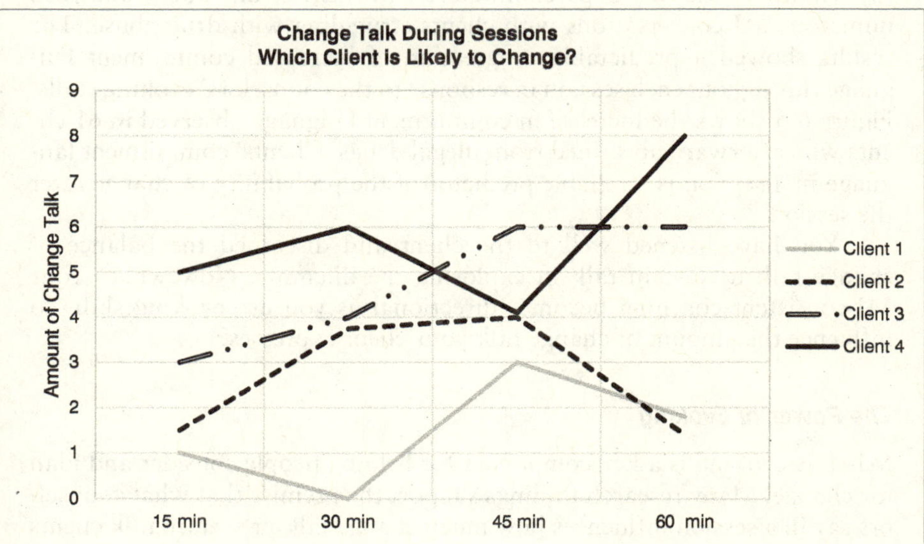

FIGURE 6.4. Change talk during sessions. Which client is likely to change?

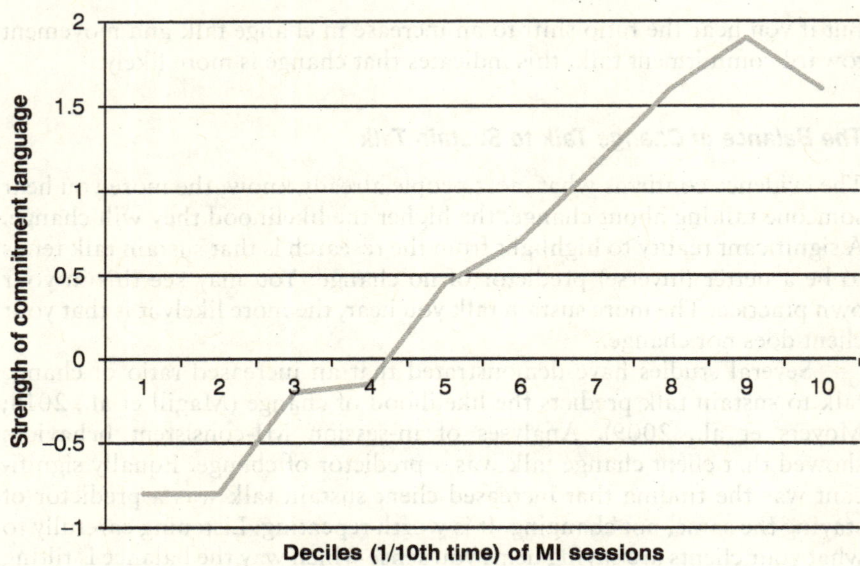

FIGURE 6.5. Strength of commitment language during MI sessions. Negative values represent commitment to continue drug use; positive values represent commitment to stop drug use. Data from Amrhein et al. (2003)

Another study by a psycholinguist (Amrhein et al., 2003) analyzed numerous MI conversations with clients struggling with drug abuse. The results showed a predictable progression of increased commitment language throughout each session in response to the counselors' evoking skills. Figure 6.5 shows the increase in commitment language observed in 61 clients who afterward abstained from illegal drugs. Clients' commitment language in a session is a reliable predictor of the probability of change after the session.

You have listened well to the client and discerned the balance of change talk to sustain talk in exploring the dilemma. Now what? Your MI-consistent coaching becomes directional as you use evoking skills to influence the amount of change talk your client expresses.

The Power of Evoking

MI-style evoking is a key component for helping people consider and plan for change. Many research findings support the premise that what counselors say in a session influences how much change talk or sustain talk clients express. (We assert this is also true for coaches.) The end goal of evoking is to draw forth your client's motivation for change and their ideas for how to make it happen. The motivation includes how important they think the change is and their perceived ability to achieve what they desire. Hearing one's own voice and arguments is a powerful catalyst for change. Your skill of evoking will continue in the planning task as you call forth the client's own ideas and preferences about how to proceed with the change (Chapter 13).

Before diving into the "how to" of evoking, we summarize a few important aspects to note in the evoking task.

- Remove your expert hat and instead emphasize your clients' autonomy.
- Refrain from inserting your arguments for change; avoid client reluctance.
- Shift to a directional (not directive) approach; use evoking skills to guide clients (detailed in Chapter 7).
- Invite your clients to make and verbalize their own arguments for change.
- Listen for the change statements woven together with sustain statements.
- Listen for the ratio of the change talk to sustain talk in a session.
- Evoke clients to strengthen and increase change talk and decrease sustain talk.
- Note the progression of change talk and determine the likelihood of client change.
- Listen for change talk, and when you hear it, *be ready to do* something!

Take It Further

Directions: Work with your learning community to read and discuss your answers to questions 1–4. Complete question 5 independently, then compare notes with your group.

1. What might you hear in your client's language if they are ambivalent about a particular change?
2. What is your role in the coaching conversation when you hear change talk and sustain talk? Why is it important to hear more change talk than sustain talk in a coaching conversation?
3. Complete the following statements: More sustain talk predicts _____________. More change talk predicts _____________. Equal change talk and sustain talk indicate _____________?
4. Which of the DARN statements relate to the perceived importance of a change? Which relates to a person's perceived confidence to change?

5. Read the dialogue below. Identify the client's change-talk and sustain-talk statements. What do you notice?

COACH: You want more consistent exercise, and you'd like to get back to swimming.

CLIENT: That's right. We have a community pool nearby, and it would be easy to jump in after the kids go to school. I need to swim because it's something that relieves a lot of my stress. I just don't have time for it, and I don't prioritize it. But I've always enjoyed it, and I can count it as aerobic exercise because it increases my heart rate. We get started in the morning then something happens, and I put other things first. If I skip it in the morning, then it seems too late to swim in the afternoon. Besides, I need my energy to make dinner. I can't plan my day well enough to fit this in. If I could just make a plan, that would be something I could do.

Chapter 7

How to Evoke

The word "evoking" implies *doing* something to forward your client's change process. But first, you are *being* the person your clients can trust. You demonstrate compassion and acceptance for your client, and as you actively listen, you become aware of change talk when you hear it. Once you recognize it, you respond in ways that encourage more of it. You are helping your clients resolve their ambivalence as they verbalize internal arguments they have not yet fully explored. As a wise gardener, you cultivate change talk while remembering that growth in the garden cannot be forced, it can only be nourished.

THREE SKILLS OF EVOKING

As we have already discussed, your first task is to become attuned to the sound of change talk and sustain talk. Next, instead of waiting for more change talk to come to you, you can invite more of it. Finally, you can strategically respond in ways to strengthen the change talk you heard.

Recall the general flow depicted in the MI hill of change (Chapter 6), demonstrating the sequence of what one might hear—or hope to hear—in a session: clients moving from preparatory change talk (uphill) to mobilizing change talk on the other side (downhill). Desire, ability, reasons, and need (DARN) statements are on the uphill side, the preparatory side. As the conversation continues and you use evoking skills, you expect to hear commitment, action, and taking steps (CATs) on the mobilizing (downhill) side.

The Coach Approach

Coaching is not a scripted practice, and as much as it seems easier to follow a manual, doing so runs counter to MI practices and the coaching paradigm. It is not a teacher-led walk where kindergarteners hold tightly to a long, connecting ribbon to keep them in line. On the contrary, Miller and Rollnick have described MI as a dance between coach and client. Listening and responding to your client in the moment are essential.

Donning the coaches' CAPE (compassion, acceptance, partnership, empathy) is a reminder that both partners are needed for change to occur. Clients have expertise in their own lives, and you bring a level of expertise also, although this does not mean you assume to know the answers. Evoking change talk is used not as a manipulation tool but as a way to activate clients' own motivation and resources for change.

The Skill of Attending

Change talk will be expressed by ambivalent clients and often mixed with sustain talk. When you hear change talk statements, begin mentally collecting them for later use. Take the opportunities they present to you and learn to recognize these statements as choice flowers among a field of weeds; pluck them and hold onto them. The example below demonstrates an equal amount of change statements and sustain statements. Can you hear the change talk woven between the sustain talk?

> "I need to get better sleep. I know it's good for my future health, but I really don't like sleeping more than 4 hours. Now that I'm retired, I want to start the day with a calm and rested mind. It's just that I love scrolling my phone at night, and it helps me relax."

It's easy to miss opportunities if your ear is not attuned to change talk and sustain talk. When coaches review their recorded sessions in a learning community, some are surprised at how much these opportunities are overlooked. One thing that hinders this skill of attending is when you focus on collecting too many pieces of data from the client. It can sound like an interrogation and not a conversation.

"How much do you sleep?"
"What time do you go to bed?"
"Have room-darkening shades been helpful?"
"How long have you been doing this?"

The emphasis seems to be on trying to solve a problem. The antidote is to sit back, practice restraint, and listen deeply with a curious mind.

The Skill of Inviting

Imagine a child perched on a fence, wishing for a horse to ramble over and visit. He turns to his mother and complains, "The horse isn't coming." Reassuringly she says, "Just hold out a carrot, and whistle." Evoking is a direct invitation. Instead of waiting for the change statements to start, you can actively invite your clients to express them. Bring your coaching mindset of curiosity. This parallels the ICF standards of "evoking awareness" and "forwarding client growth."

Directional Questions: DARN

Directional questions about desire, ability, reason, and need (DARN) can nudge the conversation in degrees moving forward. For example, with the client who wants (desires) to get better sleep, you might ask, "What do you *want* instead of 4 hours of sleep?" or "Why would you *want* to get 8 hours of sleep?" Questions about ability might be "What strengths or strategies do you have that could help you make this change?" "If you decided to change your sleep, what could you do to make it happen?" You might frame reason questions more directly, "You said it's good for your future health," and "What are other top reasons for you to do this?" Questions about need are prompting the clients' perceived level of importance for this change. "How important is it to change your sleep habits?"

Directional Questions: Importance/Confidence Scaling Questions

Asking scaling or ruler-type questions is one way to evoke change talk, specifically about the perceived importance of change (need) (Miller & Rollnick, 2023). To elicit a client's need you might ask, "On a scale of 0 to 10, where 0 is 'not very important' and 10 is 'the most important thing,' how important is it to make this change?" This question has some value, but when paired with the follow-up questions, it becomes a more effective way to elicit change talk. When a client gives you a number (e.g., 4), you follow up with "Why are you a 4 and not a 0?" Always compare to a lower number because the answer to this question will likely be change talk. If you were to ask, "Why are you a 4 and not a 9 or 10?" the client would respond with sustain talk. The third follow-up question to elicit more change talk would be "What would it take to get to a 10?"

You can also use scaling questions to ask about a client's perceived ability (confidence) to make a change. "On a scale from 0 to 10, how confident are you that you can do this?" The follow-up question would invite more confidence or ability statements. You can create many variations of ruler-type questions that better suit the clients and invite more change talk. See Figure 7.1 for the importance and confidence rulers.

0	1	2	3	4	5	6	7	8	9	10
Not at all important										Extremely important

0	1	2	3	4	5	6	7	8	9	10
Not at all confident										Extremely confident

FIGURE 7.1. Importance and confidence rulers.

Use your intuition and judgment about when you might want to use these scaling questions. The question, "How ready are you to make this change?" tends to assume that clients are on the far side of the hill, the mobilizing change talk side. That assumption may apply too much pressure for some people, so we suggest using the importance and confidence questions. While these techniques are helpful, we recommend using no more than two scaling questions in a conversation, as it can become tiresome.

Responding to Sustain Talk

When you want to evoke clients' desires, ability, reasons, and need for change, steer clear of questions whose answers would be more sustain talk. Early in the session, in the engaging task, you may hear sustain talk and decide to build rapport and offer an empathic reflection. But in the evoking task, avoid dwelling on sustain talk, especially if the person is still vacillating between two sides of the argument. Undesirable questions that seem to fan the flame for arguments to stay the same are:

"Why have you not made any change to improve your sleep?"
"You want to quit, but what is your favorite thing about chocolate?"
"Why couldn't you just put your phone in another room?"

However, even though you search for and cultivate change talk, you do not want to ignore sustain talk altogether. You can respectfully acknowledge it, and offer reflections, but then become intentional about evoking more change talk. Remember that your responses can influence and call forth change talk *or* sustain talk.

Double-Sided Reflections

One way to respond to sustain talk is to use a double-sided reflection (Miller & Rollnick, 2023). "You want to apply for the leadership position, and you don't want to have extra responsibility."

This reflection acknowledges the sustain talk while combining it with change talk into one statement. You serve a tray with both comments so that clients can see their competing arguments for change. Should you use the conjunction *and* or *but* when combining two sides of the coin of ambivalence? One can almost sense the anticipation for what will follow in statements using the word *but*.

> "You have the right content here. I like what you're saying, *but* . . ."
> "That's a good strategy that may work for you and a few others, *but* . . ."

The *but* seems to nullify or at least suppress what came first in the sentence, thereby minimizing the importance of what will come next. In contrast, when the conjunction *and* is used, you hear a seemingly fair standoff between two arguments in ambivalence. Clients offer both arguments, and the clear choice is up for negotiation.

> "You don't like to meditate, *and* you need a mindfulness practice for your stress."
> "You live in Switzerland with the best chocolate in the world, *and* you want to cut back on eating chocolate."

Placing the sustain talk first and change talk at the end is an effective strategy because, as Miller and Rollnick noted (2013), people usually respond to what they heard last. However, whether you place the sustain statement or change statement first is not a deal-breaker. The point is that if you pick out and respond to sustain talk more than you do to change talk, you will be steering the conversation in the wrong direction.

Take caution to avoid any hint of sarcasm, persuasion, or judgment in your tone of voice. Letting go of your preferences about the "right" choice takes a conscious effort, but it can help to avoid stirring up clients' reluctance as they try to defend their choices against yours.

Decisional Balance Tool

Listening to the balance of the pros and cons of change can reveal clients' readiness to change. If they are in the contemplation stage, juggling both sides of the argument for change and expressing equal parts change talk and sustain talk, the expected outcome is for ambivalence to persist (Magill et al., 2013). Some might choose to use the decisional balance (DB) tool so clients can collect a detailed list of pros and cons for changing and staying the same, hoping they will make a favorable decision to change. However, this tool can backfire with ambivalent clients and give voice to status quo arguments, resulting in no change.

Using the DB tool with ambivalent clients will likely perpetuate the motivation to stay the same and decrease the commitment to change (Miller & Rose, 2015). To foster your clients' movement toward change, you will turn up the volume on change talk and quiet down sustain talk (Prochaska, 1994). Later, you will learn how you might use the DB tool in situations where you want to remain neutral, such as when a client is deciding between career options or academic institutions (see Chapter 11).

Using Extremes

Another way to invite change talk is to ask ambivalent clients to describe some possible extreme consequences of their behavior. "What are the best possible outcomes if you make this change? What are the worst possible outcomes if you don't make the change?" Follow up with reflections, open questions, and asking for elaboration.

> "What's the worst that could happen if you kept drinking more wine at night while the kids sleep?"

The other extreme would be to ask about the best possible outcomes that might result from making a change:

> "What are the best results if you decluttered your office?"
> "If you decided to end this relationship, what good things might happen?"

Looking Back or Forward

Current problems can cloud the view of possibilities for a better life and bog people down in a limited perspective. In these cases, it is often helpful to expand their view by looking back to a time before the current problem existed. Clients get a snapshot and possibly see the discrepancies between the "now" and what used to be.

> "What was your life like before the limits of painful inflammatory arthritis?"
> "Think back to when you had peace of mind that you now hope to achieve."
> "How is life different for you now versus 15 years ago when you didn't have these headaches?"

If these rear-view mirror questions offer no encouragement, use an approach better suited to your client.

Another strategy is to invite clients to imagine an ideal future where they have successfully made the desired changes. Coaches often use a "magic wand" exercise and ask clients to imagine what life would be like if they could magically erase the problem.

> "If all conflicts with your employees were suddenly gone, what would be different?"
>
> "When you talk about losing 100 pounds, you become discouraged. How might you feel when you are at your ideal weight in the future? What will life be like?"

Exploring Goals/Values

Another way to cultivate more change talk is to invite clients to take a bird's-eye view and survey their larger *why*. Invite them to take stock of the values that drive them, what is most important to them, and their desires and aspirations for a better self in a better future. Clients' short-term goals or action steps make sense within this larger context of their values. As discussed in Chapter 5, taking time to explore clients' values is a good investment and will help to sharpen the discrepancy between current behaviors and clients' values and visions for their lives. (Goals are explored more in Chapter 13, on planning.)

A Pendulum Method

Pushing clients is likely to result in pushback, so instead, a successful coach masterfully evokes clients' internal reasons for change. But sometimes, clients persist in offering a list of reasons not to change and they express all of their qualms. If you hear a retort with every question you pose about change, it may be time to shift the approach. When change talk is not on the table, a pendulum-style method of reflecting some sustain talk first can open the door to then asking about the other side. Try listening to their cons first and offer reflections that create awareness of the reactance or sustain talk. Taking a neutral posture may open the door for exploration of the other side of their change arguments.

CLIENT: My doctor said I have to get better sleep, but I just can't.

COACH: What are some reasons you want to get better sleep? [*Trying to use an open question to evoke change talk.*]

CLIENT: I don't think I can do it. Maybe I've just given up getting a good sleep. [*No change talk.*]

COACH: You've struggled to get sleep. [*Reflecting sustain talk.*]

CLIENT: None of those phone sleep apps work, and no supplement I've tried helps either.

COACH: You've done all you know to do. What else hasn't worked? [*Reflecting sustain talk.*]

CLIENT: Someone told me to shut down technology and screens an hour before bedtime, but that's the only chance to catch up with people. And besides, it relaxes me. [*More reasons to stay the same.*]

COACH: Relaxing at night is important, so you're not taking away the screen time at bedtime. You've tried sleep apps and supplements. [*Brief summary of sustain talk.*] What kind of impact does your lack of sleep have on your work? [*Evoking change talk.*]

CLIENT: I push coffee all morning, and then I get nervous and anxious. To be honest, I'm not as patient with my co-workers as I'd like, and by two o'clock, I'm really dragging. [*Possible reason to change.*]

COACH: Lack of sleep limits your energy for work and impacts how you interact with co-workers. In what other areas of your life are you seeing an impact? [*Asking for elaboration and more change talk.*]

Reflecting some sustain talk first may help to open up a consideration of the other side, but be careful not to stoke the fires of a person's sustain talk, since that has a predictable negative outcome. You will only use the pendulum method if the momentum seems stalled and change talk is absent.

The Skill of Strengthening Change Talk

Miller and Rollnick candidly said, "Whenever you hear change talk, don't just sit there" (2013, p. 183). You first attend to, listen for, and collect change-talk statements. But noticing and collecting change talk is not the end goal; it's a means to an end. The third skill, strengthening change talk, involves using what you gathered and responding in ways that increase the amount and strength of the change talk.

Chapters 1 and 3 explained that MI and the coach approach are client centered. But this is not an approach where listening, asking, and reflecting exist in circular conversation in which clients lead and coaches nod in understanding, repeating what they heard. That passivity is a misconception about coaching. Instead, in this approach coaching is a forward-moving, collaborative relationship to help clients get *results* in their personal or professional lives (ICF, 2007). More than listening is required. The MI approach provides the template for *how* to strengthen change talk in the evoking task by using OARS skills to intentionally steer the boat toward the chosen destination.

Directional Questions: OARS Becomes EARS

In the engaging task (Chapter 4), you use OARS skills to build an empathic partnership with your client. In the evoking task, you strengthen the change talk by using open questions to ask for more examples and elaboration (EARS). With EARS you are exploring the change talk and using authentic curiosity to hear more about it.

> "What are some ways your job could be better?" (elaborate)
>
> "You're not happy with the fatigue you feel after eating sugar. What are other examples of what you experience after eating a lot of sugar?" (examples)

The second statement elicits the disadvantages of the status quo, which by default evokes the advantages of changing (change talk). The client may respond, "I get headaches. My brain feels 'foggy,' and I get sleepy." These are examples of reasons to change.

Directional Affirmations

Another effective way to strengthen change talk in the evoking task is to use affirmations directionally to highlight clients' strengths, efforts, and the change talk you notice. "You're pretty determined to get this weight off"; "You've debated this and have taken the time to consider what's most important"; "It's evident by your past success that once you commit, you do what you say you'll do." By using affirmations to strengthen change talk, you avoid the roadblock of giving empty praise.

Directional Reflections

Your reflections directly influence whether you hear change talk or sustain talk (Apodaca et al., 2016; Magill et al., 2019). Your task is to strategically reflect the change talk. The expected result is that clients respond with more change talk, and as this pattern continues, the ratio of the change talk to sustain talk increases, and so does the likelihood of change (Magill et al., 2018). Listen for the change talk in this coaching sample, where the client wanted help to stop drinking her nightly red wine.

> "I've had headaches my whole life, and my entire family has them, too; it's a genetic thing. I have two passions: red wine and coffee. I read that red wine is better for you than white wine, so now I have red wine at night and three cups of coffee in the morning. Of course, I need to take headache pills in the morning. It could be that wine is causing headaches, but you might as well just take the love out of my life. It's

easier to take the pain pills than to try and get to the root of what's causing these headaches. Imagine what the point of living is if you can't have wine. I'd rather have headaches. This would be very important to me, and I might think about giving up coffee, but red wine is non-negotiable."

Intently listening uncovers change statements mingled in with sustain talk. Once you recognize these, you can collect them and use them later. You are using the skills directionally by intentionally choosing what to reflect on, ask about, and summarize. The change statements in the above example are:

"I just have to figure out what's causing these headaches," "I have to take headache pills in the morning," and "It might be that wine is causing headaches." [The sustain talk that follows—"but you might as well take the love out of my life"—almost obscures the change talk.] "This would be very important to me," and "I might think about giving up coffee."

In the continued conversation below, the client offers more change talk. (The change talk statements are *italicized*.)

"Recently, *they've been getting worse*, but I think they connect to my emotions because my mom recently passed away from a heart attack. I've had a lack of sleep, and I know that links to headaches. *But I just would love to stop wine. Maybe I need an accountability partner who says, "Okay, you can't have the wine for a week." But I want to see my headaches go down from a 9 to a 3. Then it would be worth it.*"

Directional Summaries

In the engaging and focusing tasks, summaries help to connect and check in with clients to ensure mutual understanding or to bridge earlier discussions to new ones. In evoking, clients have a chance to revisit and hear their change talk, first when you use evoking questions, then when you use reflections to invite even more change talk. Each successive time they will hear themselves talking about change. MI summaries take on the unique purpose of pulling together the collected blooms of change talk and offering these as bouquets to clients. As we mentioned, you may want to offer smaller summaries—posies—throughout the session. As the conversation continues, a larger summary bouquet allows them to hear their arguments for change one more time.

Understanding *why* you might use these summaries makes it easier to know *what* to summarize. Directional summaries in the evoking task strengthen change talk by revisiting and highlighting the change talk spoken by the client. Resist the temptation to summarize everything the client said, focusing less on your skill of recall and more on strengthening your clients' change talk.

Practicing Directional Summaries

This skill takes practice. Below is a presentation of four summaries that a coach might offer in the scenario presented earlier, where the client wonders if red wine and coffee give them headaches. Read each one and decide what impact each summary might have. Which ones are MI-consistent? How might the client feel and respond to each? Why?

> *Summary 1*
>
> "You're having serious struggles with headaches right now, and they are getting worse. It might be because of your grief about your mom, and the lack of sleep doesn't help. Life is stressful enough and removing your two passions—wine and coffee—might even make things worse. You can't imagine giving them up, especially now, because they give you joy and enrich your life. You might consider giving up coffee, but you are unwilling to give up wine. Do I have that right?"

If a coach used this summary in the engaging task, the client might feel understood and that the coach listens with compassion and acceptance. The coach emphasizes mainly the emotions around the dilemma. Although this summary would be MI-compatible in engaging, it does little to move the conversation forward. This summary lacks a goal-oriented direction needed for the evoking task and may leave the client stuck in the same struggle.

> *Summary 2*
>
> "You want to stop your headaches and figure out what causes them because, even though you tried hormone medication and eating healthy, nothing has worked. You could have a genetic problem or a lack of sleep due to grief. You wonder if red wine and coffee could be the root cause, but you can't imagine life without them. They are your passions, and you'd prefer to take pain meds in the morning instead of quitting wine and coffee. But still, if you had some accountability, you might stop coffee, but absolutely not wine."

The coach includes two sides of the client's ambivalence, attempting to give equal time for both arguments. It's as if the coach is helping the client consider the pros and cons, much like one would do with the DB tool, which in this case would probably evoke more sustain talk. (As we discuss in Chapter 11, the DB tool may be effective when the coach is neutral and wants to avoid influencing a client either way.)

Notice that sustain talk is positioned last in the final sentence, which likely echoes as the most pronounced—and memorable—of the two statements. One can predict the expected result of this summary will be for the client to remain ambivalent. This summary is not helpful in the evoking task where you want a forward direction toward a specific goal.

Summary 3

"You have serious headaches, and I think you're in denial about the issue. Emotions and lack of sleep make things worse, but the real problem is the wine. Every night you drink wine, you wake up with a headache. At first, you said accountability might help you stop the wine, but then you said you'd rather have headaches than give up wine. This sounds like an unhealthy dependence on wine. Do you agree?"

This summary is accusatory with a judgmental and even parental tone. The summary attempts to persuade the client by presenting the "facts" as evidence, possibly hoping that the client will hear and, with sudden insight, slap their forehead and say, "Ah, now I see!" But instead, the likely result would be reluctance and more arguments to stay the same. Furthermore, this summary may also cause a rift in the relationship, described as discord (see Chapter 9).

Summary 4

"You're really struggling with headaches, and it is important to find out what's causing them. You took positive steps to check your hormones and eat a healthier diet. Grieving has caused you to lose sleep, and you wonder if those emotions are making the headaches worse. Even though having a glass of red wine in the evening and three cups of coffee in the morning brings you a lot of joy, you wonder if those could cause headaches. You don't want to give those things up, but you might consider it for a time just to test the theory. What other things might you try?"

This summary is an MI-consistent summary. The change talk is picked from a field of blooms and presented to the client as a bouquet. The last open question asks the client for even more flowers. Although all the summaries presented above are about the same length and take approximately the same amount of time, only Summary 4 is appropriate for the evoking task. This summary will likely strengthen change talk and ensure that a forward direction toward the goal is underway. Using EARS skills moves

BOX 7.1. How to Evoke Change Talk

Attending to change talk

- Listen carefully.
- Collect the change talk.

Inviting change talk

- Listen carefully.
- Use directional questions: DARN.
- Use scaling questions or ruler questions.
- Explore extremes.
- Look back or forward.
- Explore goals or values.

Strengthening change talk

- Use EARS—questions asking for elaboration and examples of the change talk.
- Affirm change talk and the strengths it implies.
- Use directional reflections (to evoke more change talk).
- Use directional summaries (to reflect the collection of change talk).

the conversation in the direction of the goal. See Box 7.1 for a review of evoking change talk.

So, how do we answer the paradoxical questions revisited in Chapter 6, "If this is a client-led approach, what role do I play in supporting clients movement toward change?" In engaging, you built a relational, working alliance that demonstrated unconditional positive regard for your clients, where they felt safe enough to explore their hopes and dreams and dilemmas. Afterward, you collaborated to find a focus and destination for the work ahead. In evoking, you actively promote and evoke clients' expressions of change talk and allow them to talk themselves into change.

But to further explore the second question, "How can I help someone if I shouldn't tell them what to do?," you may wonder if giving advice or information is warranted. On the surface, it seems counterintuitive in MI-consistent coaching, since you do not want to jeopardize the client's autonomy and self-discovery. However, skillful advice-giving can be consistent with MI practice and coaching, and we will explore this technique in Chapter 8.

Here is a conversation with a client who is referred by her physician to address diabetes and hypertension caused by weight gain. The doctor prescribed a food plan as a weight loss intervention before the next step of increasing the medication. In this example, Bailey, the client, is in her third session.

COACH: Hi Bailey, welcome back. What did you accomplish last week that you're pleased with? [*Open question.*]

CLIENT: Honestly, not much. After my failure the week before, I lost confidence to try anything. Besides, it was my 40th birthday, and I was not going to ruin it by staying on a diet just because my doctor ordered it. It's too hard, and I don't want to set myself up for failure again.

COACH: You don't turn 40 every day! Happy Birthday! That's something to celebrate. [*Reflection, engaging.*]

CLIENT: Thanks! I had a great party. I rented the gym and invited some friends to join me for a rowing workout. They all came, and we had a fantastic time racing each other, then I invited them back to my house afterward. I'm getting ready for a marathon rowing challenge this month, and I asked for their support to help me stay accountable. I didn't overdrink the night before, so I felt strong. One friend stood up, clapped for me, and said, "It's good to have a friend like Bailey, who wants to work out on her birthday."

COACH: Wow, Bailey, that's a creative way to celebrate! You're taking care of your body and connecting with friends at the same time! You even inspired them. [*Affirming.*] What was your reaction to the toast? [*Open question.*]

CLIENT: I got teary-eyed because that's the kind of person I want to be. They texted me the next morning and said, "Hey, don't forget you said you would row 10,000 meters today." So, I went to the gym and got it done. [*Client hints at her broader vision of her ideal self.*]

COACH: You *did* accomplish one of your goals by not overdrinking during your birthday celebration. What helped you achieve such a challenging goal? [*Affirmation, evoking open question.*]

CLIENT: I think because I made a promise on social media, and to my friends, to you, and to my spouse that I would do this. So, I did it. I'm thankful to everybody for holding me accountable and supporting me because that was really important to me. But I have to be honest and tell you I have not eaten well this week at all. I didn't keep a food diary; I ate things I shouldn't have, and I definitely had too much alcohol. *But I did increase water, and I rowed every day. I'm trying to do a little bit better than I did the day before.* I can't figure out why I can't just jump right back in and get on track. I don't know what's happening. *I think the goals I set 2 weeks ago were probably unrealistic for my age.* It's not reasonable to lose 10–12 pounds every month.

[*Open question prompts client self-discovery.*]

[*Sustain talk mixed with change talk. Evidence of ambivalence around the prescribed food plan.*] (Change talk is in *italics.*)

COACH: You've made progress in many areas that seemed easy to you, yet some areas are very hard. [*Reflection, empathy.*] What do you want to focus on in today's session? [*Guiding the focus.*]

In the initial part of the session, the coach engages with the client and demonstrates active listening and empathy. The client is highly motivated to reach her self-imposed goal of rowing a marathon within the month. Yet she is not making progress toward the goals for weight loss from her doctor. The coach listens well to the ambivalent statements and the client's strategies to accomplish her "really important" goal.

CLIENT: *I want to focus on going forward,* but I don't want a deadline. *I have a goal and dreams, and aspirations,* but a deadline automatically stresses me out, and *I need to try and work hard to release that stress. That stress puts weight on me and makes it such that I can't focus. That's kind of what I would like. I need help to set a goal* rather than a deadline. And you know, I have a

[Client and coach worked on a vision during the last session.]

[*Self-discovery, change talk.*]

couple of trips coming up, and before, I was like, "*I want to be 30 pounds lighter by that date.*" But I'm not going to be there, and I put so much pressure and stress on myself to do that, so when I don't do it, I kind of spiral. [*Sustain talk mixed with change talk.*]

COACH: For you, a deadline is a measurement of perfection. [*Amplified reflection.*]

CLIENT: Yes, absolutely! One of my favorite quotes is from Robert Frost, "The pursuit of perfection is a recipe for depression."

The conversation has been somewhat circular to this point as the coach ensures that rapport is established. The coach provides the space for the client to express her ambivalence within a safe, nonjudgmental space. The client's mingling of change statements and sustain statements indicates that the task of evoking motivation may be in order.

COACH: I notice you put hard boundaries and deadlines around your rowing. What's the difference between this and your other weight loss goals? [*Directional reflections.*] [*Directional open question.*]

CLIENT: That's a great question, and I'm not sure I know the answer. Rowing is the one thing that's taken priority over everything. I was supposed to go out with friends tonight to a concert, but I've got to row tomorrow morning, and if I go out tonight, that's probably not going to happen. It's certainly not going to happen to the standard it needs to happen for me to continue to train.

COACH: That standard is pulling you forward past those competing priorities. You flourish in your social connections, and yet you are forgoing that—which is a high value in your life—to finish this goal of preparing for the marathon. [*Exploration of goals/values.*] Something about this particular goal is so important to you that you will temporarily make that harder choice. [*Directional affirmations.*]

CLIENT: *I think what you just said—temporarily—is the key to getting my goal. My weight loss goal is not temporary; it's for the long term.* And I can't cut my friends out of my life for the year it's going to take for me to do this.

COACH: You can't see yourself setting deadlines and boundaries around your weight, and on the other hand, you're successful with rowing because you set a hard commitment. You've got support, and you can see the deadline in the near future. This is your sixth marathon. You have one mindset around your diet and another one around rowing. [*Directional double-sided reflections.*] [*Directional summary.*]

Notice the shift toward a more directional use of the skills in this conversation since the client expresses ambivalence with change talk and sustain talk. The coach begins to invite and strengthen change talk by using directional EARS. The evoking may occur over several sessions or transition toward planning in a single session. The client's readiness to change will determine the pacing of the session, but the coach guides the journey forward by shining a light from stone to stone to cross unfamiliar murky waters.

CLIENT: So, it's interesting because, you know, in three *weeks that I did really well on this eating plan, the one week that this worked was when I put it all together. I did the meditation, the food, and the exercise in one week, and that was the week I had the most success. So, I feel like the exercise part is crucial. For me to have a good positive mindset to do the eating, it has to go hand in hand with other things.* [*Client insight and discovery.*] [*The entire response is change talk.*]

I struggle with putting eating and exercise together with the mental, spiritual, and emotional parts of it. To wrap it up in one big package and make it work for me.

COACH: So, you've seen that it does work when it's a package deal. *[Reflection, restraint.]*

CLIENT: Yes, and it has to be a package deal.

COACH: It's a three-legged stool; if one leg breaks, the whole stool comes down. Like when you accidentally had gluten, you got so frustrated that you chucked the whole plan. *[Reflection, a metaphor to look back.]*

CLIENT: Yeah, I'm still not recovered from that.

COACH: When you have goals for rowing, but something gets in your way, what is your mindset or strategy for moving past that setback? *[Directional open question.]*

CLIENT: I just go back and do it again the next day. It's interesting because it doesn't translate to the rest of my life, and I didn't get that until you just said it.

COACH: I have an observation; may I share it with you? *[Asking permission.]*

CLIENT: Sure, please do.

COACH: Fun and creativity were two values you listed as "very important." How might it be helpful or important to bring those into the food plan goal? *[Explores values and strengths.]* *[Directional open question.]*

CLIENT: *It's very important*! And now that you've pointed it out, *I think I need to bring creativity into that part. I never thought of it that way. You know this weekend my spouse and I are going to cook together. We love to do that.* I stopped cooking because he's mostly vegan and vegetarian, and I can't come up with any way to make something creative the way I used to. *But I found a recipe online that we're going to try tomorrow night, so there's an opportunity for us to be creative together and see what works and what doesn't work and then maybe tweak it. Maybe—not maybe—definitively, that* *[Activation, commitment language.]* *[Stronger commitment language.]*

seems to be what I need to do: bring creativity and fun into this way of eating rather than making it an albatross that just hangs around my neck.

COACH: This albatross; its perfection around the diet. Let's pull out and think about what's drawing you toward this weight loss journey. What's really driving that boat? [*Reflection of meaning, directional open questions for a larger vision.*]

CLIENT: I think *I'm tired of fighting the same battle every single day.* It's exhausting, you know? *I just want to see people I haven't seen in a while, but I have gained more weight, which is embarrassing. I'm tired of hiding in my house, and it's frustrating and depressing to have to fight the same thing.* That is what I'm going to fight forever until I die, and thinking of it that way is super overwhelming. [*An abundance of change talk.*]

COACH: And yet you are here. What made you show up for coaching, for your therapist, and for your spouse? [*Affirmation and directional questions asking for elaboration.*]

CLIENT: *I guess I can't lose hope. I can't give up. I'm not a quitter.* I know it's weird because I quit for little pieces of time, and then *I come back. I wish I could shorten the amount of time between quitting and coming back. But I want to give myself grace. I think I haven't completely quit because I'm still growing. I'm still seeing you and trying to do some positive things, so I haven't just shut everything off, which is what I would have done.* [*Ability language.*] [*Self-affirmations and building confidence.*]

The client's preparatory change talk has shifted toward the mobilizing side of the MI hill, and commitment language is increasing. The coach guided the conversation by inviting and strengthening change talk. The client's readiness to change seems to be high, and the increase in change talk indicates that it's time to begin transitioning to the planning task as the natural next step.

Take It Further

Directions: Work in your learning community to read the coach's reflections below. Then, determine which of these are MI-consistent reflections you might use in the evoking task.

a. Many other things like grief can impact your sleep and cause headaches.
b. You're trying hard to figure out the cause of these headaches.
c. You need to find the cause of these headaches, but wine and coffee enrich your life so much that you'd rather have headaches than give up wine and coffee.
d. It seems your headaches are a genetic problem, somewhat out of your control.
e. Giving up wine or coffee would be worth it if your headaches decreased.
f. Having some accountability would allow you to test your theory that wine or coffee is the cause of your headaches.

1. Which of the reflections will likely elicit more change talk? Explain why.
2. What might be the result of using reflection "c"? Explain why.
3. Which reflection will likely result in sustain talk? Explain why.

Chapter 8

Sharing Information and Advice

Sharing information and advice is a hot topic in coaching. We recognize that it can be jarring to hear that you will leave your expertise aside and let clients find their own solutions. Since coaching is not built on the deficit model, you act on the assumption that clients have the resources within themselves to design and achieve their goals (Williams & Menendez, 2015). So, where does that leave informing or advising as a coaching skill? Coaches new to this way of helping might conclude either they tell clients what to do, or they sit back while clients figure things out on their own. In fact, usually, neither of those approaches is particularly helpful.

"Antinomy" describes a contradiction between two equally valid truths (Oxford Languages, 2022). While it is true that clients are experts in their own lives, and you are not in the information delivery service, it is also true that clients want and need information to help them move forward. MI methods serve as a link for this antinomy, creating the conditions for sharing information and even advice in a way that preserves clients' self-discovery and choice. Your expertise in the coaching process and your use of the guiding style are vital in this journey.

You may need to share information, advice, or your intuitive insights throughout the coaching process to advance client growth. Early on in coaching, clients may need information about the coach and client roles. After that, you might offer information as the search for a focus gets underway. In evoking and planning, information can become a catalyst for choosing what to change and how best to create sustainable momentum toward change. This chapter describes the MI method for sharing information and advice within the coach's scope of practice. We present a few scenarios where sharing information is more likely to be needed and

TABLE 8.1. Sharing Information in the Four Tasks

Engaging

- As you understand more of your clients' dilemmas, you may hear hints about what they believe is most important to them.
- In the initial session, they may ask your opinion on which direction to take, "what to do," or "where to start."
- Sharing information may be a part of helping clients consider how the coaching agreement will help and what to expect from the coaching relationship.

Focusing

- In the focusing task, sharing information can help clients narrow their choices and find a clear focus.
- Collaborate to harness the clients' experience and wisdom about what has worked for them in the past.
- Clients uncover the collected wisdom and knowledge, then seek to understand and use this information to move in their chosen direction.
- In this way, it is more of an interchange than a one-way delivery of information.

Evoking

- In evoking you elicit change talk to strengthen clients' motivation and commitment to change.
- At this time, you might share information that helps them consider both sides of their ambivalence and imagine ways to close their intention/behavior gap.
- You also may find that you need to address misinformation.
- Although clients might need or want information and advice to help prepare for and imagine a way forward, you hold fast to the skills of listening, reflecting, and asking open questions.

Planning

- In planning, you continue to evoke clients' ideas and solutions for change.
- As clients "try on" strategies for achieving goals, they might benefit from your information, advice, or, sometimes, personal disclosure.
- You do this while keeping clients' needs as a top priority.

explore some best practices for offering information. Specific MI strategies are explained, and broader guidelines are offered for effective practice. See Table 8.1 for a quick reference on ways to share information in each of the four tasks.

SHARING INFORMATION AND ADVICE IN A GUIDING STYLE

Good tour guides discover what attractions and destinations the travelers want to see and then give the information needed to navigate the journey and glean the most from the experience. These guides walk alongside, pointing out interesting facts and relevant things to consider, neither leading the way nor walking behind on their own journeys. In the same manner, as a guide, you point to the chosen destinations and offer information when needed so clients can make the best choices for their journey.

As we mentioned earlier, MI is on a continuum between a purely person-centered approach (Rogers, 1980) and a more directive intervention and treatment model. Although the two converge and overlap at times, MI strikes a midpoint, guiding, which includes some components of each. In MI-consistent coaching, you refrain from the impulse to fix people, something Miller and Rollnick call the "fixing reflex" (2023). A collaborative approach allows sharing of information and advice while preserving the personal relationship that is critical to the success of this method. As we have said, in our approach the MI methods and guiding style infuse the entire practice of coaching. Because MI is perfectly congruent with offering information and advice, coaching is also (Miller & Rollnick, 2023).

As guides, you assume clients are experts and creators of their own lives; they are creative, resourceful, and whole (Kimsey-House et al., 2018). Your expertise in the coaching process equips you to help clients "discover, clarify, and align with what (they) want to achieve" (ICF, 2022). Since the focus is client discovery, self-generated ideas, responsibility, and accountability, you share information to support that growing competence. Therefore, sharing information and advice is secondary to that facilitative process. Informing and advising are used succinctly and judiciously since clients possess the best answers within themselves (Williams & Menendez, 2015).

COACHING SCOPE OF PRACTICE

Coach training programs highlight the distinctions between coaching, psychotherapy, and other helping professions. They urge coaches to stay within their scope of practice, since these boundaries make it easier to determine when and if other professions would be a better fit for clients. Furthermore, ICF's core competency 1 states that coaches should clearly communicate the distinctions between coaching, consulting, psychotherapy, and other support professions (we provide a link to the ICF core competencies at *www.guilford.com/lanier-materials*). When you clarify and share these distinctions with your clients, you uphold the integrity of coaching. The masterful coach may combine advising, mentoring, consulting, and teaching elements but keeps the distinctions in view to remain in the scope of practice. Advisors give specific strategies for solving a particular issue based on their expertise, which the learner may or may not follow. Mentoring is a long-term relationship where mentors offer their experiential wisdom, direction, and guidance related to the learner's career. Consultants are experts who work on a short-term basis to find problems, prescribe, and implement solutions. Teachers define learning outcomes and focus instruction to help learners clarify, organize, and prioritize new information (Marcdante & Simpson, 2018). Table 8.2 might be a useful reference to remind you and your clients about these distinctions.

These roles overlap and meld to influence the coaching practice, depending on the circumstance, but here again, the issue is less about what information is shared and more about *how* it is shared. When you inform, educate, or advise, the overarching expectation is to avoid encroaching on clients' autonomy (Deci & Ryan, 2013). As you seek to determine the nuances of how to offer information and guidance within your scope of practice, recall that research has repeatedly found that the single most essential ingredient is the relationship between the helper (coach) and the client (Norcross & Wampold, 2018).

The NBHWC further clarifies the scope of practice for coaching (2020):

> While health and wellness coaches per se do not diagnose conditions, prescribe treatments, or provide psychological therapeutic interventions, they may provide expert guidance in areas in which they hold active, nationally recognized credentials and may offer resources from nationally recognized authorities such as those referenced in NBHWC's Content Outline with Resources . . .
>
> [Coaches] support their clients in achieving health goals and behavioral change based on their clients' own goals *and* [our emphasis] consistent with treatment plans as prescribed by individual clients' professional health care providers.

The clear message is that although clients may need information and education, a coach should offer it within specific parameters. You can give expert guidance in areas where you hold dual qualifications, and when this is not the case, you may use other credible resources. As a health coach, you may work collaboratively with the client's health care provider, which usually requires educating the client. Another parameter is the quantity of time dedicated to informing. The NBHWC advises coaches to spend at "least 75% of each session devoted to coaching facilitation and not education" (National Board of Medical Examiners & NBHWC, 2022a).

How do you offer information without crossing the boundaries of the coaching contract, which defines the coach and client roles? Coaching is not a top-down, information-dispensing method to fix clients' problems, yet sometimes a bit of information is helpful. Since the primary aim is client learning, discovery, and growth, the type of help you offer is different from a therapist or educator. MI-consistent methods will help you stay within the scope of practice and ensure that clients remain actively engaged and autonomous in the process.

TABLE 8.2. Distinctions of Coaching versus Expert Roles

Item	Coach	Advisor/consultant	Mentor	Teacher
Focus	What's working, use of core strengths and values	What's wrong, what to fix, and reducing problems for specific outcome	What skill and character to develop for specialized field	What knowledge, skill, attitude (KSA) to provide for learners
Expertise	Clients—experts in their lives; coaches—experts in coaching process	Experts in targeted performance or skill	Experts in the same field, having experience with success to share	Experts in prescribed learning objectives for the learner
Control	Client-directed, coach co-discovers answers in a working alliance	Top-down flow, advisor/consultant directed, supply answers	Expert-driven, mentors supply answers	Expert-driven, teachers supply answers
Strategy	Inspires, advocates, and facilitates client learning, discovery and insight to find solutions	Gives advice, prescribes and directs based on norms for performance	Transmits information based on mentor expertise and experience	Dispenses knowledge, educates, implores, assesses acquisition of KSA
Time	Time-limited, current	Single or few sessions	Long-term, future	Time-limited, current
Results	Active engagement, co-creation, empowerment, effective action	Possible low compliance, resistance, and new problems	Possible low investment or ownership of change	Possible low engagement or broader use of KSA

WHEN EDUCATION IS NEEDED

You can educate your clients—minimally—while also empowering them to find their own solutions. The collaborative, trusting relationship sets the template for informing and advising without provoking unnecessary sustain talk, discord, or disengagement (Brehm & Brehm, 2013). Before outlining *how* to share information and advice, we present some typical circumstances where coaches may need to educate or advise.

Prescriptions in Health Coaching

Health practitioners refer patients to coaches and may give them prescriptions for lifestyle or dietary changes. They may expect you, the coach, to fill in gaps of knowledge to help their patient understand the prescribed changes. Although an exchange of information may be necessary, you know that clients need more than this to close the intention–behavior gap and arrive at growth and sustained behavior change. Consider how to respond when a client has this mistaken assumption:

> "My doctor told me I had to change my eating so I can get my blood sugar under control. If you could give me a diet to follow and tell me what to do, I think that's all I need."

Performance Goals in Life Coaching

Employers or other organizational leaders may refer people who need to improve performance and may expect you to focus on skill development or work-improvement strategies. Coaches should do this minimally and avoid intruding on client autonomy (Jordan, 2022). You want to engage and promote self-discovery, not shut it down.

> "My superintendent told me to improve student achievement, and I don't know what else I can do. She probably assumes you'll tell me some good strategies."

In this case, the client needs information about the coach's role and the client's responsibility for active engagement within the coaching alliance.

Competing Goals

Your client's goals may differ from their health practitioner's protocols or their employer's work performance goals. In these cases, you, as the coach, learn the delicate balance of addressing both. How is this done? Skillful coaches can shift and offer information or advice while remaining neutral

BOX 8.1. Sharing Information in Health and Wellness Coaching

In the current medical model, there are often gaps between what the physician prescribes and what the patient does. On some level, the client may need clarification of the facts in order to comply. However, as Leigh-Ann Webster, executive director for the NBHWC, said, "The challenge of implementation isn't always that the person is unaware of what to do" (2022). She reiterated what we all experience: Roadblocks get in the way of making that sustained change. Good health coaches can help fill this gap by taking time to help their clients figure out "what's getting in the way of success" and then helping their clients create roadmaps to achieve success. Forward movement will require sharing necessary information or advice in the context of a collaborative relationship where the client's autonomy is a carefully guarded component.

in favor of the client's best interest. You balance these goals while staying keenly aware of the client's stage of growth, their current level of understanding, and their needs and desires. Since goal progress depends on client readiness, address the third-party goals within a context of respect for the client's choices and unique pace of growth. (See Box 8.1.)

> "My doctor gave me this nine-step plan, but there's no way I'm going on that Elimination Diet right now. I want to try some of the other eight steps first. Can you give me some advice?"

Client Expectations

If clients enter coaching with an assumption that your job is to tell them what to do, they are not entirely mistaken—you will, of course, inform them within your role as a coach. But as we said, providing information is not your primary job. Clients do their own research and work. You uphold your contract agreement, which specifies your roles and responsibilities, while also taking this opportunity to clarify the collaborative nature of coaching. Coaches often take time to do this at or before the initial session.

> "My HR department told me to learn team management skills. I assume you'll give me some training, and then I'll be on my way."

When education is needed, you fill the gaps so clients can craft a way forward toward success. But informing and advising are secondary to the process of client self-discovery and awareness around their motivation, desired outcomes, and goals. The collaborative coaching relationship is the foundation, the fertile soil where clients' ideas and possibilities for change can germinate and grow.

A STRATEGY FOR SHARING INFORMATION AND ADVICE

The MI way of exchanging information safeguards clients' autonomy to engage as creative problem solvers, and it empowers them to exercise the freedom to explore what suits their strengths and needs. You share information as a collaborative exchange among equals, and the relationship's success depends on the trust built in the partnership.

When you share information that implies a suggestion for how and what to change, it becomes advice. Your client may appreciate and even ask for advice, but that is tricky; the benefit depends on how the message is received. Offer information and advice with neutrality, without conditions or expectations, to minimize possible resistance. (Coaching with neutrality is specifically addressed in Chapter 11.)

The general principle is to respectfully get permission before sharing anything. Of course, if a client *asks* for information or advice, they are giving permission by virtue of the request. Once permission is granted, find out what a client already knows and zero in on what interests them most. Offering relevant information raises attention and responsiveness and promotes an engaged and responsive client. Dumping buckets of information or advice on the table would likely get you the opposite.

Knock Before Entering

Ask permission before barging in with information, suggestions, or advice; being invited is better than being perceived as an intruder. Avoid persuading, which may inadvertently apply varying degrees of pressure. Psychological reactance theory says that a threat to or loss of freedom motivates the person to restore that freedom (Brehm & Brehm, 2013). Here are examples of appropriately asking for permission.

- "Would you be interested in hearing what experts say?"
- "Which things on this list from your superintendent can I clarify for you?"
- "Would it be helpful if I offered some other ideas?"
- "If you're interested, could I share what has worked for other clients?"

When clients ask for information or advice, they are giving permission. Here are some examples.

- "What do you think I should work on?"
- "Would you have some recommendations for me?"
- "Can you suggest some ideas for reducing stress?"

While these questions signal an invitation, frame your response with the awareness that your clients are resourceful, and they most likely have ideas of their own.

Speak with Respect and Honor Autonomy

People already possess freedom and will exercise the right to take or leave what you have to say, so respectfully acknowledge that freedom when offering information or advice, thereby avoiding defensiveness (de Almeida Neto, 2017). A simple strategy is to preface what you say with respectful language. Here are some examples.

- "This may not apply to you . . ."
- "When you decide what to do . . ."
- "You may have already thought of this . . ."
- "Your opinion is what matters most . . ."

In the spirit of authenticity, you may not want to ask for permission when you have something you feel is essential to your client's progress. In this case, the MI skill of honoring autonomy runs parallel to the ICF competency 7, "Evokes Awareness," which states that the coach shares—without attachment—"observations, intuitions, concerns, thoughts, or feelings and invites the client's exploration" (2019b). When sharing something you feel is necessary though not asked for, offer it without condition and honor a client's choice to consider it or not.

- "I'm not sure if this is important to you, but I want to offer some clarity."
- "I have a few concerns about your plan. You may not share this feeling, but I want to explain what bothers me about it."
- "I'm observing a pattern and wonder if you notice it, too."

Offer Options and Space

Choosing among several options empowers people and makes it more likely that they will stick to their choices. But offering options one at a time can prompt people to refute each one, even in their internal dialogue. Though this rebuttal is typical of ambivalence, coaches should avoid stoking that fire and evoking sustain talk. You want to encourage the exploration of possibilities, not squelch them. For example, the client is a mother who wants to make more time for herself and her kids by getting organized at home. The client responds to each option, citing reasons why each idea will not work for her. (Notice how the client rebuts each choice with more sustain talk.)

CLIENT: Do you have any suggestions for how I can get my house organized?

COACH: [The coach gives options one at a time; client responses are in *italics*.]

- Maybe you could hire someone to help you. (*"No, I can't afford that."*)
- You could make a checklist of the things you need to do and order them by which is most important. (*"No, I hate lists, they make me feel pressured."*)
- What about tackling one room at a time to throw out what you don't need? (*"No, I would get too overwhelmed with a whole room."*)
- You could get a friend to help. (*"No, I'm too embarrassed to let anyone see my mess."*)

Instead, below, the coach offers several options without pausing between each one, thereby reducing pressure to accept or reject each idea. Clients are more apt to feel the freedom to consider choices when you present a smorgasbord of options from which to choose.

COACH: There are many possibilities for getting organized at home. Could I share some things that other clients have tried? (*Client agrees.*) Some people hire a personal organizer to come to their home and help sort it out. Others like to check off items from a list. Some want to focus on one room at a time before moving to the next space, and others get motivated if they have a friend working alongside them. Which, if any, of those things appeals to you? Can you think of other options?

CLIENT: Yeah, those are some good ideas, but really, as I hear you talk about it, I probably need to throw stuff away first and start in one room and work my way from there. Maybe I could pick the easiest room first.

This respectful way of interacting reduces any inherent pressure to receive information, especially advice.

ASK–OFFER–ASK

Unsolicited advice can be hard to accept. Sweeten the bits of information and advice with a good dose of listening and respect to make your offering easier to sample. The MI ask–offer–ask (A-O-A) method provides information while keeping clients engaged, motivated, and in the driver's seat of their lives. A-O-A is not necessarily a linear process but can become a circular, rhythmic, and collaborative volley between you and the client, where ideas, information, and even advice enrich the conversation and positively influence the change outcomes. The most important thing is always to begin and end with the client's perspective.

Ask

One ASK is directly asking for permission to offer information, which ensures that you stay in the guiding style and out of a directive posture.

- "Could I share a few ideas with you?"
- "Would it be helpful if I shared something about . . . ?"
- "Would you like to know more about that?"

A second good starting point is to ASK what clients already know. Their prior knowledge, efforts, and experiences can uncover possible gaps in their understanding and prevent you from telling them what they already know or have already tried.

- "What kinds of things have you already tried?"
- "What do you already know about increasing student achievement?"
- "How much do you already know about stress management?"

You may also find it helpful to ASK what clients *want* to know. We find it is often quite different than what the coach believes they need to hear.

- "What are you most interested in learning about this topic?"
- "What types of information would be most helpful with this new goal?"

A client asking about which foods balance blood sugar does not necessarily want to hear the mechanism for how the pancreas delivers insulin to the cells. Clients are more likely to receive what they consider most relevant and important.

The A-O-A cycle can also get started when clients request that you *tell* them what to do.

- "I just need you to tell me what to do to manage stress. I don't know where to begin, and it's all too confusing. Could you give me some resources?"
- "Can you tell me what strategies I can use to get my student achievement scores higher?"

But before diving in with a list of "stress management strategies" or "best practices for teaching," first, remember the overarching goal of client self-discovery and self-regulation. Prevent inadvertently nudging clients toward a passive role and remember that telling clients what to do—even if they ask for it—could potentially undermine their autonomy.

You may consider that clients had previous helpers who doled out prescriptions and protocols; therefore, they may expect the same from coaching. "I have a problem, and you can help me by just telling me the information I need." As previously mentioned, this assumption can become a learning opportunity before or during the initial session when you discuss the coaching contract.

Additionally, discern whether the "tell me what to do" request implies low client confidence or a genuine lack of knowledge about the issue. The seasoned coach also listens for other concerns beneath the surface of the request. Tuning in to those unspoken issues before jumping in with information will safeguard the collaborative working alliance.

Offer

The second part of the A-O-A cycle is OFFER and comes after you ask—and wait for—an answer. MI-consistent practice is to offer small doses and refrain from opening the firehose and dousing your client with extended streams of information. Ask permission, then offer the chunk of information. The key here is to offer only a little bit at a time.

Ask

The third ASK of the A-O-A cycle is inviting a client's responses to what you offered. You can ask what they think or feel about the information or advice and check in on their understanding. In a typical dialogue, as clients become accustomed to the check-in, they may offer their responses before you ask. As we said, this becomes a circular exchange rather than a linear one.

- "What's your reaction to this?"
- "What about that interests you?"
- "What things are you still wondering about after you hear that information?"
- "How does that information suit your situation?"

The A-O-A cycle can happen within one session or several times within a session, and in some cases, it can be an ongoing process over time, as in the sample below.

COACH: Your administrator asked you to meet with me about raising student scores. What questions do you have about that?

[*Ask for what the client wants to know.*]

CLIENT: None, really. I need you to show me what to do to. Could you give me handouts with some best practices for raising achievement scores?

COACH: Sure, but first, I'd like to hear about what you're already doing that you feel is working.

[*Strengths focused. Coach asks for the client's prior knowledge and current awareness.*]

CLIENT: Well, that's just it. I thought I was effective and doing my best, but apparently, the data say my struggling students aren't achieving like they should.

COACH: You don't see eye to eye with the administrator's directive.

[*Complex reflection. The coach wonders if this is low confidence, lack of knowledge, or both?*]

CLIENT: Yes and no. As we say, the data don't lie. I obviously need to learn something I don't know, but I promise I've been doing all that I know how to do.

COACH: What might be most important for you to learn?

[*Client autonomy, and an indirect request for skill development. Possible low confidence.*]

CLIENT: To be honest, I'm struggling with classroom management. If I could get my students more engaged, I think that would make a big difference in their learning.

COACH: And you believe learning better classroom management skills will boost student engagement.

[*Reflection, without judgment.*]

CLIENT: I know it would.

COACH: And that's where you'd like to start.

[*Respectful language and honor client choice.*]

CLIENT: Yeah, could you first see what's happening in my classroom? I mean, I have so many great ideas and lessons, and lots of students are doing well. But I think there's something missing with some of them. They're not paying

[*The client feels safe. The client's tone has shifted, and the client offers an area of possible study.*]

attention, so they miss a lot of content. Maybe you could tell me what you see?

COACH: Okay, how about we schedule an observation for next week? You can target some things you want me to observe, and afterward, you and I can research and come up with a few specific strategies you might want to try. What do you think of that? [*Partnering.*] [*Coach sets the pattern of A-O-A.*]

CLIENT: That's a fantastic plan! I can't wait to talk to someone who sees what's going on and knows what I'm talking about. My administrator says, "improve scores," and he doesn't really have the time to help me.

COACH: I sense relief and maybe more confidence. [*Affirmation.*]

CLIENT: (*laughing*) I guess you could tell I was a little discouraged about being told to work with a coach, and I thought you were going to mandate another new thing from the district that I had to implement.

COACH: You're an extremely busy teacher with a mound of demands. My job is to help you decide what you want to achieve and then partner with you to plan how to get there. I'm the expert in the coaching process, but you're the expert in your classroom and your life. [*Acceptance, affirmation, and a small bit of information about the coach's role.*]

Offering Information and Advice

Carefully Correct Misinformation

When clients have misinformation (particularly around a health and wellness topic), first prioritize what they want and need to understand. Ask permission before clarifying the information, and remember that clients are more receptive when you have a trusting relationship. Avoid jumping in too quickly to correct clients' false assumptions or misinformation since this may become a catalyst for sustain talk and even discord (see Chapter 9 for more on discord).

COACH: Your doctor wants to get your blood sugar under control, and he told you to increase the nonstarchy vegetables. Which of those vegetables have you tried so far?

CLIENT: I'm eating a lot of white potatoes since that's a vegetable.

Tempering any urge to set the client straight will help avoid reactance and disengagement. Tug on the hem of your coaches' CAPE and remember that your primary purpose is not to correct clients but to cultivate change.

Offer Only Relevant Information

Receiving permission to talk about a topic is not a license to ramble on and shift the conversation away from your client. Offer only what benefits the persons in front of you, what is relevant, and what suits their unique needs. Though you may relate to the client's dilemma, stay on topic and avoid diverting the focus away from what is relevant to the client. Your conversation is based on a coach-client relationship, not on a friendship. A chat between friends may go something like this:

FRIEND A: I'm having a hard time getting everything done at work. I need a time management course or something.

FRIEND B: Yeah, I've been under so much stress, too, but I do morning meditation now, and I'm much better. My husband said he used to walk on eggshells around me, but not anymore.

FRIEND A: I need to learn how to manage my time. I can't find time for it all.

FRIEND B: You should have seen me. I was on a handful of pills for stress, then one day, I just said, "You have got to start taking care of yourself." I guess I just dug down deep and figured out what I had to do.

FRIEND A: (*long pause*) That's good. Maybe I'll look online for time management help.

When Friend B inserts her narrative, the conversation shifts away from Friend A's topic of time management, and the chat runs on parallel planes as two monologues. You have probably experienced similar conversations with friends over coffee where both of you enjoyed a renewed camaraderie and connection. Coaching is not a chat between friends; it's a strategic conversation fashioned in the best interest of clients, prioritizing their needs and keeping a laser focus on what is most important and relevant to them.

Self-Disclosure

Self-disclosure is one way to share information, but like advice, its helpfulness depends on the approach. Self-disclosure can be seen as being authentic or genuine with oneself, understanding and then communicating the "observations, intuitions, concerns, thoughts or feelings" to clients (ICF, 2020b). This kind of communication will likely spark a common chord between you and advance the relationship (Rogers, 1980). It can deepen your connection with clients and allow them to see you as a fellow human and credible partner. Authentic disclosure also models a way of being for clients, who will need to embrace authenticity and transparency when taking responsibility for crafting their lives (Williams & Menendez, 2023).

MI-consistent coaching focuses on clients' experiences and best interests, not yours. It is not necessary to share every thought you have with clients, nor to remain objective and withhold anything personal. MI—and coaching—is a balanced approach where you may share something that may be helpful.

Sometimes it's appropriate to share your personal experiences, genuine feelings, and intuitions, and Miller and Rollnick (2013) offer a few questions as tests to determine when this might be warranted. First, "Is it true?" The honest story is the best, though the coach does not necessarily need to tell the whole story. "Is it harmful?" and "Is it helpful?" are two additional tests. Even though you may have a strong opinion, consider whether it comes across as criticism. In addition to the benefits already mentioned, self-disclosure can answer client questions, such as "Have you ever had a chronic illness?" And you can affirm your genuine appreciation for a client's discovery or effort with a simple statement, such as "I feel personally inspired by your effort on this."

Keep It Brief; Be Concise

Choose what is most important to offer, especially if the information might stir strong emotions. Consider a client's stage of change, what they already know, and any possible gaps in understanding. Clarify things and make mental notes of what you need to address later, and when you do address those things, keep it brief and concise. No matter how pertinent, a long list of information can cause clients to become overwhelmed or disengaged.

Use Common, Everyday Language

Using familiar language that your clients can relate to is essential, especially in health and wellness coaching, where it would be easy to slip into technical-sounding "coach-ese." Take the opportunity to connect to your clients with speech that meets their level of understanding and experience.

Below are examples of words or phrases to avoid, with some suggestions for using everyday language after the double slash (//).

- Your optimal vision of health and well-being // Your dreams, purpose, meaning in life, and ideas for your best self and future
- Your values // What is most important to you? What drives you?
- Mindfulness // Becoming aware of the present moment without any judgment
- Saboteur // The inner critic
- Triglycerides // Fats in the blood
- Myocardial infarction // Heart attack
- Hypertension // High blood pressure

Use Language That Honors Autonomy

Autonomy-honoring language is nonconfrontational, avoids the use of shaming or scare tactics, and is not prescriptive or directive (Clifford & Curtis, 2016). Here are two examples—one that is directive and the other that honors autonomy.

CLIENT: I know the doctor told me to change my diet, but since the medicine keeps my blood sugar level, I think I'll keep my diet the way it is.

COACH A: You forget what we've talked about. Even though your blood sugar numbers look normal, you have high insulin levels. That means your pancreas is working too hard and wearing down. I'm afraid you're just delaying the inevitable disaster. You've got to stop eating the way you do!

Coach A is scolding and using inflammatory speech to scare the client into compliance.

COACH B: May I share a concern I have about this? (*Client agrees.*) You were on board with your doctor's prescription for dietary changes when we talked last week. I'm wondering, what has changed your mind?

Coach B uses respectful language to share concerns and slightly nudges the client to revisit their goals.

Calm the Hurried Mind (Emotional Contagion)

Does the following scenario sound familiar? You listen to clients and sense their urgency to change their situation, to end suffering, and quickly move from the "now" toward "not yet." You feel a strong desire to help them, so you start sharing information in a rapid-fire style. It's no wonder that clients might then experience feelings of frustration and become disengaged.

Emotional contagion is the phenomenon that describes the transference of emotions between two people. In the above situation, the coach's strong desire to help and the possible sense of urgency may interfere with the client's need to process ideas (Boyatzis et al., 2019; Hatfield et al., 1993). As Boyatzis and colleagues said, "Our brains are hardwired for picking up on the emotions of others around us" (2019, p. 71). Joseph LeDoux (2002) documented that this process happens in about 8 milliseconds, but the good news is this rapid contagion can also be positive. You can manage your emotional tone in a session and help ensure clients (and you) work mainly in a calm, parasympathetic state. In this renewal mode, clients are more likely to be open to new ideas, people, and positive emotions such as joy, gratitude, and curiosity (Howard, 2015).

By first mindfully tending to your emotions, your desire to help clients can become a positive contagion, like a cooling salve on a burning wound. Enter with a calm and unhurried presence and use the MI model to offer information within this context. People are more likely to imagine and plan for change within a relaxed and supportive relationship.

Focus on the Person, Not the Data

In the instant information world, masterful coaches intentionally resist the urge to overexplain or overinform. A well-intentioned push to "help them see" often gives the impression that the client's role is to passively receive information.

Repeating yourself or speaking louder does nothing to help people understand a foreign language. Understanding what your client needs and wants at the moment requires you to lay aside assumptions and truly listen. As much information, experience, and advice as you possess, you know that your clients are complex humans, not data banks. What you have to offer is most helpful when your clients actively engage in receiving and making meaning of the information. You, as a sage coach, will provide information that fits clients' unique perspectives.

Reframe with a Positive Message

Our brains receive and cling to the negative far more than the positive, so it's best if you reframe hard-to-hear information in a more positive light. Clients may face harsh realities, especially in the context of health and wellness coaching. Inspire hope and convey your belief in your clients' completeness. Pleasantly package the hard facts with a sense of hope and optimism. Note the difference between these two examples:

- "If you don't learn to manage stress, you're going to develop more complicated issues in the future."
- "When you manage stress, you are helping your body to heal."

Refer to What Others Do

When you discuss information that implies action, refer to what others have done and remember the caution to avoid giving one idea at a time. Remaining neutral will prevent the "fixing reflex" and confirm your commitment to honor clients as *the* experts in their lives. Your expectations, conditions, or biases can spark reluctance and, as we have said, stir client rebuttals. A posture of neutrality invites clients to explore ideas in the form of change talk and opens the door for them to explore their own choices.

> "Some clients in your situation start gradually weaning from sugar first, and others jump in and cut it out on day one. What makes sense to you?"

Coaching Sample

This client came for coaching and requested that the coach "Just tell me what to do." This is the first meeting.

COACH: You mentioned in your Welcome Packet forms that you want to know how to eat better for your health.	[*Engaging and reflecting to show understanding.*]
CLIENT: Yeah, I need to eat better, so if I knew what I was supposed to eat, I would do it. Give me a diet or something; tell me what to do.	
COACH: It can be frustrating not to know what to do.	[*Active listening, empathy.*]
CLIENT: Right!	
COACH: First, would it be ok if I reviewed our roles in the coaching agreement? (*Client agrees.*) As you know, I'm not a nutritionist and don't prescribe. I could offer information and point you to some resources. I'll ask questions to help you find answers, and when needed, we can create solutions together. How does that sound?	[*The coach educates the client on the coach/client roles using the* A-O-A *model.*]

CLIENT: Yeah, I understand. I'm here to get the information, and then I'll be ready to go.

COACH: What do you understand about your role as a client?

[*The coach first asks what the client knows.*]

CLIENT: I mean, I'm here to change, right? It's simple, really. I show up, you tell me what to do, and I do it.

COACH: Yes, you'll be taking responsibility for making the changes you want. As you become more self-aware, you'll be curious and open to suggestions or new possibilities. How does that resonate with you?

[*The coach is aware of the potential misunderstandings and uses A-O-A to clarify the roles, which both parties have signed in a contract agreement.*]

CLIENT: Yeah, I remember that from the contract. So, you'll give me my orders, and I'll follow them.

COACH: I can offer some ideas and support you along the way. As your guide, I want to be helpful and not waste your time. So first, share with me what you already know about healthy food.

[*The coach uses respectful, autonomy-honoring language in an A-O-A approach to find out what the client knows about the topic of healthy food.*]

CLIENT: I know what's *not* healthy. I mean, my roommate and I eat out every meal because neither one of us cooks. Fast food and pizza aren't good, and soft drinks have sugar. But I don't know what else to eat, and I don't have much choice because I don't cook, so I have to eat the wrong stuff.

COACH: And you want the right stuff, the healthy food.

[*The coach reflects change talk.*]

CLIENT: Yep, I mean, my dad has all kinds of health problems, and he says that I'm just like him, so I'm probably headed for some diseases in the future. I'd feel better if I ate better, but like I said, I need someone to tell me what to eat.

COACH: First, I want to understand what would be helpful. Would you consider taking an imaginary trip to the grocery

[*The coach uses autonomy-honoring language.*]

store with me? (*Client nods.*) Imagine you and I walked into your favorite grocery store. We're standing there with our grocery cart, and our job is to buy healthy food. Which food would you put in your cart?

[Another ASK. The coach lays the groundwork to model the style of interaction, emphasizing client engagement and autonomy.]

CLIENT: I don't really know.

COACH: (*Silence, waiting.*) There's a lot of confusing information out there. But let's say we're in the store, and I asked you to point to where we should shop first. Where would you point?

[The coach resists the "fixing reflex," and defers to the client's resourcefulness.]

CLIENT: Okay, I guess I'd point to the perimeter of the store because I know that most healthy foods are around there, but the packaged stuff and less healthy things are usually in the middle aisles.

COACH: Yes, that seems to be the way things are arranged. And just so we're on the same page, what kinds of food are on the perimeter of the store?

[The coach evokes confidence by affirming and ASKs about prior knowledge.]

CLIENT: Well, I guess that's where they keep the vegetables and fruits.

COACH: It sounds like you already have a good foundation for choosing healthier foods like vegetables and fruits. What other information would you want or need to help you eat better and be healthier?

[The coach affirms the client's knowledge, and checks in with another ASK to see what the client needs and wants.]

CLIENT: Yeah, I'm not giving myself enough credit. I probably know what to eat, but if I had a list of vegetables to choose from and some recipes or ways to prepare and cook them, that would be a good place to start. Have you got some ideas for me?

COACH: Sure. Would you like to have a simple food plan that other clients have found helpful to get started?

CLIENT: Yea, as long as it has recipes.

COACH: It has recipes and menus. I'm curious, though, since you don't cook, how do you want to use the recipes?

CLIENT: Well, it's clear that I have to start cooking unless I can find good restaurants. But like I said, I eat mostly fast food, and the vegetables are minimal. I need to learn some basic cooking skills, right? I think my roommate and I could get into that. It might be fun.

COACH: I have a few suggestions to help you get started. (*Client nods.*) Some clients learn one or two recipes at a time so they can repeat that throughout the week. Others subscribe to a food service that delivers the ingredients with directions for cooking the meal. And some use a simple formula for the dinner meal where they pick a protein, a vegetable, a salad, and maybe some fruit. Which, if any, of those appeals to you?

[*"What others do": The client has previously asked, which is permission. The coach offers options without pauses.*]

[*The coach uses autonomy-supporting language.*]

CLIENT: Well, maybe I could go ahead and order that meal service and then work on learning just one recipe this week.

Take It Further

Directions: Work in your learning community to read and answer the questions below. Access Handouts 8.1–8.3 (online at *www.guilford.com/lanier-materials*) to answer questions 2, 3c, 4, and 5.

1. Refer to Table 8.2, "Distinctions of Coaching versus Expert Roles." Consider the various roles presented in the table and include any others you have experience in.
   a. What are some possible challenges for you in sharing information and advice?
   b. Give some specific examples of how you would use the A-O-A method for offering information or your intuition and observations.
2. Refer to Box 8.1, "Sharing Information in Health and Wellness Coaching." Discuss how a health and wellness coach could share information in a way that guards the collaborative relationship.

3. Imagine that you have a client who says, "Just tell me what to do."
   a. What factors would you consider before answering?
   b. What are possible cautions to be aware of as you coach?
   c. Locate Handout 8.1, "Telling Clients What to Do." Read what one coach has to say in response to this question. With your group, discuss other insights or ideas you may have.
4. Locate Handout 8.2, "Distinctions and Dealing with Emotions in Coaching." Discuss some practical ways you, as a coach, can address emotions and remain in a coaching role.
5. Locate Handout 8.3, "Additional Resources for Dealing with Emotions in Coaching." In your group, share your experience with dealing with emotions in coaching. What are any new insights you have?

Chapter 9

Evoking and Responding to Discord

Some ambivalence is natural when you evoke clients' "what," "why," and "how" about a change they seek. Considering the sources of this reluctance can help you frame a supportive response and avoid inciting client reactance. This chapter clarifies the subtle but essential differences in sustain talk and discord and offers MI-consistent ways to respond.

In Miller and Rollnick's first edition of *Motivational Interviewing* (1992), "resistance" was used when describing the behavior of more difficult clients. Meanwhile, they felt uncomfortable with that term because it implied clients were to blame for their ambivalence. As MI practice grew, studies confirmed that clients' resistance—expressed as sustain talk—increased or decreased depending on what counselors said in the interview (Magill et al., 2018). As we have noted, what you say in response to clients' language can influence the amount of change-talk or sustain-talk statements you hear from them. So, the question is, is the sustain talk you hear an expression of the clients' normal, internal pro-versus-con argument, or is it a response to what you say? Those are two different things.

In the second edition of *Motivational Interviewing* (2002), "rolling with resistance" was introduced to suggest how practitioners should respond versus react to clients' ambivalence. However, the growing unease with "resistance" persisted since it implied a pathology versus something normal. Finally, in the third edition (2013), Miller and Rollnick abandoned "resistance" altogether, since they realized that most of what had been labeled resistance was merely sustain talk. When you unlink sustain talk from what helpers think of as resistance, the only thing left is what MI calls "discord."

Ambivalence, being of "two minds," is a normal experience of simultaneously conflicting motivations. The good news is that when you hear ambivalence, the client is at least considering a change. As we said, weighing the cons of change is not a disorder (Miller, 2022). The client may be reluctant about a goal: "I just don't want to change the way I eat." Or their hesitancy may indicate an internal struggle with two equally difficult choices: "I'm committed to caring for my mother in the nursing home, and I can't do it. My job demands my full attention, at least for now, and I feel guilty."

When clients say, "I don't want to," "I can't," "there's no reason to do it," and "I see no need to," those DARN statements are about the change topic. But other statements may point to something else:

- "You haven't heard me."
- "It's not a question I think you should ask."
- "Well, what would you do if your wife did that to you?"
- "You didn't tell me I shouldn't do that."

Those statements echo something besides ambivalence about a change goal. The word "you" is a clue; it sounds the alarm that something has changed and points to some disharmony between the client and you and the relationship itself. This is discord. Sustain talk points to the problem or focus, but discord is about the relationship.

Not all discord is terrible, and rapport can be built, broken, and rebuilt again in a very short time. Sometimes, you might find that discord allows you to reaffirm clients' efforts, character strengths, or wavering confidence. It may also be an excellent time to become aware of and strengthen your coaching skills of attention and careful listening.

Preventing discord is always an aim, but once you hear it, there are ways to heal it. In most relationships, when one partner begins to climb the ladder of contention, the other person can ascend the other side of the ladder and respond, escalating things, or stay on the ground and soften the matter. We discussed ways to respond to sustain talk in Chapter 6. This chapter is about softening discord so you can reharmonize the relationship in a spirit of compassion and partnership. The general strategy when you sense discord is to resist climbing the ladder with a "fixing reflex."

COACHES' CAPE: COMPASSION, ACCEPTANCE, PARTNERSHIP, EMPOWERMENT

All the strategies for responding to discord flourish only within the context of the MI spirit, which we introduced in Chapter 3 as the coaches' CAPE. As we explained, we took the components of the MI spirit and arranged them in the acronym CAPE. You, as a coach, will wear this CAPE as a reminder of the coach approach and the *way* you show up with your client.

Clients come to you because either they believe or someone else believes they need another person, a partner, to help them change. This partnership is the safe place where clients can be vulnerable and voice the pros and cons of their inner whispered dialogue, where you listen without judgment. Within this safety, they trust you to compassionately hear their inconsistent thoughts, or what may appear to be a head-versus-heart debate. "I need to stop shouting orders and let my employees see that I'm more approachable" (head), but "I get so frustrated when they don't pay attention to the details of the task" (heart).

Underneath the sustain talk, you may hear your client's yearning to answer the universal question, "Will this person [the coach] really understand me?" A compassionate response can open the door for clients to explore and resolve their ambivalence, but a "fixing reflex" can shut down the discussion or move things in the wrong direction. You may understandably feel a profound responsibility and urgency to help clients know what and how to change. But when you argue for the pro side of change, with a degree of pressure, you risk inciting a counterpoint response from the client in favor of staying the same (Brehm & Brehm, 2013). Pressure, persuasion, or any implied threat to personal choice can tilt the balance and cause clients to take a firm stand on the opposite side, reasserting their autonomy. This fixing reflex can incite discord. In the example below, the helper champions change talk—the pros of change—while the client responds with increasing sustain talk.

COACH: If you keep working this way, you risk losing your health.

CLIENT: Yeah, but so far, I'm okay. The doctor's referral note is a suggestion, not an order.

COACH: So far, but what about later? How much longer can you work 14 hours a day?

CLIENT: My job is demanding, especially with all these deadlines. I'm performing at a high level, so my new supervisor added to my responsibilities. There's no time right now to take care of myself.

COACH: Your health is more important than the job.

CLIENT: But you don't understand what I have going on right now.

Start with acceptance, with the assumption that people have choices, and remember that attempts to steer them away from their freedom can invite reactance. "You cannot keep working this way" is not true, and what you mean is something different. Acknowledging each client's autonomy can avoid a potential push-back defense and reassertion of their power to choose. You should, in essence, open the door and say, "You can do what you want." Yes, this may feel risky, but you honor their autonomy and believe clients can find their own best solutions with your skillful guidance. One of the powers of coaching with MI is that your clients express their ambivalence without judgment or threat to their autonomy.

Offer a choice without the slightest hint of sarcasm or disbelief in your voice. Practice saying, "It's your choice to eat what you want," sarcastically or dismissively, then practice saying it in a supportive and respectful manner. Notice the sound of your words. Which one conveys respect for your client's autonomy to choose? Here are a few other responses that can demonstrate your respect for a person's choice:

- "Which food you decide to reintroduce next is up to you."
- "With all the options you have, I wonder what you'll choose."
- "You get to pick the option that works best for you."

REFLECTIONS FOR SUSTAIN TALK AND DISCORD

We described several types of MI-consistent reflections in Chapter 3. Here, we review those and then expand on some that you might want to add to your toolbox. This discussion applies to sustain talk *and* discord since most general strategies are the same, except that you can ask for an apology in discord.

Regarding discord, an ounce of prevention goes a long way, but once you hear it, the first option is to acknowledge it and then reflect on it in a straightforward manner. Here are some *simple reflections:*

CLIENT: They don't understand me. I don't know if you understand me either. [*Discord.*]

COACH: You're not feeling understood, and that is important for you. [*Reflection.*]

CLIENT: I don't really need to learn stress management right now. [*Sustain.*]

COACH: Stress management isn't your top priority right now. [*Reflection.*]

CLIENT: My boss scolds me in front of my peers. I can't produce with that kind of pressure. [*Sustain.*]

COACH: You want more support from your boss so you can be more productive. [*Reflection.*]

Another MI response is an *amplified reflection,* where you turn the volume up on what the client said. As you magnify and overstate their words, this often invites clients to reconsider what they actually mean versus what they said or what you reflected. Often, it's within this exchange that clients get to sort their thoughts and test them to see if they are true. Hearing the words as if through a megaphone can unmute a discrepancy between their highest values and their current behavior or thinking. Keep your CAPE on when you do this, and speak from compassion, avoiding sarcasm or any tone of ridicule. Here are some examples of amplified reflections to sustain talk and discord.

CLIENT: She didn't invite me to the meeting, per usual. [*Discord with others.*]

COACH: She never includes you and ignores your input. [*Amplified reflection.*]

CLIENT: I have the gene for heart disease, so changing my lifestyle won't help. [*Reluctance.*]

COACH: You have no control over your genes. There's no point in even trying. [*Amplified reflection.*]

CLIENT: I'm too busy to exercise since I work full-time. [*Sustain talk.*]

COACH: It's impossible to exercise as long as you're working full-time. [*Amplified reflection.*]

CLIENT: You don't understand. I can't focus on the diet because I'm trying to figure out my life purpose. [*Discord and sustain talk.*]

COACH: It's impossible for you to find your life purpose and work on health at the same time. [*Amplified reflection to sustain talk.*]

MI emphasizes accurate empathy and using reflections to come closer to fully understanding what clients mean. Likewise, you match your client's energy and emotions with a warm tone and become attuned to their emotional state (NBHWC, 2022). However, to soften sustain talk and discord, it can be effective to use reflections that understate (or overstate) the client's intensity to shift them toward self-discovery. Like amplified reflections, understating what the client says can be a catalyst to usher them to reconsider and express their emotions about a situation more accurately.

CLIENT: I'm offended that my husband says to drop my volunteer jobs. [*Discord with others.*]

COACH: You're a little bothered with him. [*Understating.*]

CLIENT: Bothered? I'd say I was angry with him. He just isn't listening to me!

The third type of reflection we discussed is the *double-sided reflection* (see Chapter 7). Here, you insert a client's sustain talk as a counterbalance to the pro side of their ambivalence that you heard earlier in the conversation. This client is experiencing happiness in her new marriage but is sad about gaining weight.

CLIENT: You don't understand how long I've waited for this marriage. I'm finally happy, so I eat comfort foods. [*Discord, sustain talk.*]

COACH: You're happily married, so you eat your favorite foods, and at the same time, you've gained weight since the wedding, which distresses you. [*Double-sided reflection.*]

As a reminder, a good strategy for a double-sided reflection is to begin with the client's discord or sustain talk and end with their change talk. The conjunction "and" is a better choice since "but" tends to negate or devalue what came before it.

OTHER STRATEGIC RESPONSES

In addition to the general strategy to respect client autonomy, acknowledging and reflecting discord in a straightforward way, you may find these additional strategies helpful in softening sustain talk and discord.

Apology

If discord is a relationship problem, whether you nudged it or not, you can initiate the reconnection by offering an apology.

CLIENT: You don't seem to understand my problem.

COACH: You're right. I'm sorry. I'm listening now and want you to help me understand.

CLIENT: I'm angry you skipped over my strong emotions around this issue.

COACH: I apologize for moving on too quickly. Your emotions are worth exploring, so let's spend more time on that.

Align with Them

Sometimes, despite your attempts to evoke awareness of "what is" and "what could be" your clients remain reluctant. They persist in their sustain talk or discord—temporarily—and the possibilities of change are not yet apparent. One MI strategy is aligning with them, wrapping arms, and walking in accord. As you agree with them (though not entirely), this can exert the right energy to evoke change talk.

- "You're right. You can't change your bad genes, no matter what you try."
- "Maybe you have to keep working 14 hours a day, even if your health suffers."
- "I see your two options: Eat what you want and be happy, or diet and be miserable."

Here again, when you reflect on what they said, a measure of self-regulation is called for to avoid a "fixing reflex."

Reframing

Home decorators insist, "The picture frame makes all the difference!" You can create a dark and moody tone or a light and whimsical one just by switching out frames. The same principle applies to softening discord and sustain talk. As a coach, you help clients become aware of choices in their lives, and reframing is a subtle way to offer the client a different perspective on the situation.

Reframing is the skill of getting a new view of something. Skillful coaching helps clients place their thoughts or stories in a new context and see the positive side of what was previously considered a roadblock (Williams & Menendez, 2015).

CLIENT: My principal is stressing me out with all these extra jobs, and I don't think I can do it.

COACH: Your principal has a lot of faith in your ability. [*Reframing.*]

CLIENT: This diet food is gross. You've taken away all my joy! I guess I have to learn to eat like this for the rest of my life. [*Sustain talk, discord.*]

COACH: Yes, it can take time to develop a taste for vegetables. I wonder how you might use your strength of creativity to bring joy back to eating. [*Acknowledge and reframe.*]

Shifting Focus

Sometimes discord is not about the relationship between you and the client but may stem from other connections in their social circle or a wider group of experts who prescribe or demand change. The discord with others, or even with you, may spark blaming. Recall that this is one of the traps we discussed in Chapter 3. An MI-consistent approach shifts attention or blame away from one topic or person to another, more positively focused one. A client may say, "The school superintendent is unreasonable, and she's the source of my stress. Are you saying I should accept that as part of my job?" You might respond, "Blaming your superintendent is a natural tendency. How about you and I spend time planning ways to get the work–life balance you want?"

DISCORD IN THE FOUR TASKS

Why is discord a concern, and how can you know if it's present? Discord is a significant concern because it indicates a rift in the relationship, and this rift negatively impacts subsequent change. A large body of research demonstrates that the quality of the relationship—the working alliance—is the best predictor of psychotherapy outcomes (Safran et al., 1990; Luborsky et al., 1983). This finding is relevant to coaching as well.

As a coach, if you listen intently, you can hear the tones of friction in your coach–client relationship in the same way that even nonmusicians wince when they hear an orchestra or a choir slip out of tune with each other. Discord might sound like defending—"I'm not at fault here"—or outright opposition—"You haven't been listening to me." Another sign is when the client interrupts you—"Wait, wait, that's not the way things are for me." A more subtle form of discord is the nonverbal signals of disengagement that your client presents, such as looking away, crossing arms over the chest, or being inattentive or distracted.

Discord can originate from several sources, but it can also stem from the coach's emotional state or attitude. You may feel a sense of urgency or impatience because of third-party referrals or sponsors. Emotions may be triggered and start a cascade of internal chatter, "How can this client lack any self-awareness?" or "How will I explain to the principal that this teacher needs more support and time to make all those changes?" While you are busy managing the discord within yourself, you may have stopped listening to your client.

Discord in Engaging

As you and clients launch into the engaging task, it's not uncommon for them to rumble against what other experts have directed them to do or change. They may have a long list of reasons why that prescription or performance directive will not work for them. Some clients are new to coaching and may initially feel defensive, hoping to avoid a previous experience when they simply took orders and had no choice. "I'm not what he thinks I am; I'm not a sugar addict!" or "She sent me here because she thinks I'm disorganized on the job. I know how to plan, but I also need to be spontaneous and creative."

Although it's essential to be aware of discord in the beginning, client change is not predicted by the level of commitment and motivation at the start. Instead, the observable pattern of increased motivation throughout the session or sessions predicts change (Amrhein et al., 2003). Remember, you have the power to influence what happens next, and MI has proven to be an effective way to turn down the thermostat on anger or defensiveness (Waldron et al., 2001).

Discord in Focusing

A woman comes to you with a prescription from her doctor to exercise more. You assume that her focus will be on the goal of planning exercise into her day, so you start in that direction. But when you hear, "You don't understand, I have five kids!" you may have walked into the "premature focus trap" and incited discord. Pushing too soon for a focus that clients may not yet agree with can undermine a nurturing partnership.

Discord in Evoking

If you engaged with your client and have an agreed direction for the session, expect sustain talk to emerge in the evoking task as a natural expression of ambivalence. But, if you nudge too quickly toward a direction when the client is not quite ready, discord can surface and is a predictable consequence of the fixing reflex. The example below demonstrates a client who feels pushed and could benefit from more time in the evoking task.

COACH: You've talked about how important movement is to your overall health.

CLIENT: Sure, it's important, and I know what I should do, but it's hard to fit it in.

COACH: It's hard, but it sounds like you're ready to commit. What ideas do you have?

CLIENT: Yea, it's important. But I'm not so sure I'm committed just yet. [*Reluctance.*]

COACH: Let's review the reasons you need this. How will you build commitment? [*Pushy.*]

CLIENT: Are you hearing me? I have five children, a full-time job, and community obligations. I hardly have time for my kids, and you're pressuring me to plan for exercise. [*Discord.*]

Discord in Planning

You may hear discord in the planning even after successfully engaging, focusing, and evoking task (see Chapter 13 for more details on the planning task). It can be tempting to become more directive, add details to the action step, rush the timing, or offer ways for the client to stay accountable. The MI spirit—the coaches' CAPE—should blanket the entire process from beginning to end and remind you to remain collaborative and use a guiding posture.

The common thread among all these sources of discord is a crack in the relationship, which is often a result of a clash between the client's ambivalence and the coach's fixing reflex. Sustain talk and discord need not be an alarm for you but can become an avenue for discovery as the two of you rewrite the dance steps. When you hear discord, instead of reacting, you can shift the dance in a new direction.

Coach, you can witness the suffering, the rumbling, the sustain talk or discord and respond or react to it. Your relationship is the container, the safe place where clients voice their arguments, where they dare to argue, dream, and hope aloud. Your calm responses, reflections, or even softly provocative inquiries are best delivered in the context of your compassionate guidance. The masterful coach handles these tensions in a way that empowers clients to navigate beyond their sustain talk or discord and make progress.

Here is a portion of a session with a woman referred to coaching to manage stress. Peppered throughout her language is sustain talk and discord.

COACH: What would you like to focus on today?	[*Open question.*]
CLIENT: This all started with me talking about some symptoms with my doctor. He said to manage my stress and see a coach to get help. But before I could make the appointment, I was ordered (*air quotes*) by my husband and a friend to do something that felt totally unrealistic. I wish people understood what I have going on in my life. I'm here so you can help me cut out things in my life, stress less, or something like that. But I have a lot going on, and I just have to accept it. Now's not the time to quit.	[*The client expresses discord.*] [*The word "ordered" hints that she feels pressure or pushed by others.*]
COACH: Okay, other people think stress is your primary concern, but you disagree.	[*Reflection, acceptance.*]
CLIENT: Well, the doctor wants me to manage stress, and everyone else is an expert on how I'm supposed to do that.	[*She seems to feel misunderstood.*]

Yes, stress is a problem, but the answer is not to stop doing some things that I have to do. [*Discord with others and implied discord with the coach.*]

COACH: So stress is a problem, but not *the* problem. [*Complex reflection, a guess.*]

CLIENT: Well, I'm not saying I don't have stress. The doctor's probably right that stress could cause some of my symptoms and hormone issues. But my sister, husband, and friend think I should spend 10 minutes a day doing something just for me. And they want me to cut back on some of my responsibilities in my community. They don't get it; I can't cut back anything now. [*Change talk followed by sustain talk. This is an example of reactance. She pulls the opposite way and expresses sustain talk.*]

COACH: Spending 10 minutes on yourself doesn't fit your life now, and you can't drop your responsibilities. [*Reflecting sustain talk, aligning.*]

CLIENT: Exactly! This makes no sense in my life. I mean, no offense, but you don't know me that well or what I've got going on in my life. So, working on stress is not a priority; it's not the major thing. [*She hints at blaming the coach, and she brings discord from outside to this session.*]

COACH: You're a busy and responsible person. Can you tell me more about your life so I can understand? [*Reflection, sincere curiosity and empathy, open question.*]

CLIENT: I have five kids, work full time, and volunteer in my close-knit community. If I stop for "me time," there are a lot of things that will fall apart around me, and it's not realistic. I mean, "me time," really? That sounds self-indulgent and an excuse to ignore responsibility. People suggested that I take the kids out of their after-school activities, which is definitely not going to happen; I want well-rounded kids. [*Sustain talk.*]

COACH: You certainly have a lot going on. You've got your family, your job, and all the other commitments for your community. There really is no time to take care of yourself. [*Aligning, and amplified reflection.*]

CLIENT: Well, it's not that I have zero time; it's just that I spend my time doing so much for other people. You have no idea. Do you have kids at home? [*Discord.*]

COACH: No, it's just my spouse and myself.

CLIENT: I'm working all day, and then at night, I'm on the run with kids' activities and games. What should I do, just let them take care of themselves? Asking me to stop doing some things is unfair and unrealistic. [*She's arguing with others, not the coach.*]

COACH: Yeah, there are many reasons to be stressed! [*Reflection, refocus the topic.*]

CLIENT: What do you mean by that exactly? There are many reasons to be busy, but that doesn't mean I'm stressed. It's just part of who I am, and it's me. [*Argumentative tone and discord.*]

COACH: I'm sorry. It looks like I may have misunderstood. I thought you said your family asked you to cut back on some things to help with your stress. [*Apology.*]

CLIENT: Sure, I get it. I just don't want people to assume I don't love my family or my job, or my community because I'm stressed. *They* don't stress me out; they're my joy! For someone to tell me to pause my life for 10 minutes and pull kids out of their activities, well, that is totally unrealistic.

COACH: This is a very hectic time . . . [*Empathy.*]

CLIENT: I'm telling you, just thinking about this makes me stressed. I go to the doctor to talk about my symptoms, and now everyone tells me to do something for myself. Nonsense! I'm sure you can see why I'm so frustrated. [Interrupting.]

COACH: Sure. To you, it feels like the focus is on the wrong thing here, and all this talk about cutting back only makes you more stressed. [*Reflecting sustain talk, empathy, softening discord.*]

CLIENT: Yep, I'm definitely more uptight now that I have one more thing on my "to-do" list. (*Laughing*) [The client relaxes and sits back in her chair.]

COACH: What's it like to experience that feeling of being uptight in your day-to-day life? [*Inviting change talk, by looking at what is not desired.*]

CLIENT: When I have time to notice, to stop and think about things, I think it has a big impact on me. Obviously, that's why I'm here, or why others think I should be here.

COACH: Tell me more about that impact. [*Open question for elaboration on the change talk.*]

CLIENT: Well, it's more about being uptight about things than the stress. Now that I say that out loud, I guess they're related. Maybe I get uptight with everything I have to do, and then that feeling moves into areas of life. [*Client begins to consider an alternative perspective.*]

COACH: What do you notice when you stop and think about other areas of your life? [*Evoking elaboration of change talk.*]

CLIENT: Honestly, when the kids are in bed, I finally get a break. I wash my face and get a chance to look at myself in the mirror, and I don't like what I see. I look too old for my age, my hair is thinning, and I'm gaining weight around my belly. I have acne, which is strange for someone in her mid-30s! [*Perspective shift.*]

COACH: And you think being uptight has played a role in all that. [*Reflect possible meaning, a guess.*]

CLIENT: Yes, I think it's got something to do with that, but I guess it's also about how I feel inside, how unhealthy and hyper I feel. That's kind of what I talked to the doctor about, all these symptoms. It makes sense that being stressed out can do something to your mind and body. I've heard there's a stress hormone, right? And it gets all messed up if you stay stressed all the time. Am I right about that? [*Client is aligning with the coach, and trust is building.*]

COACH: Yes, when we stay stressed for long periods of time, it's called chronic stress, and that isn't good for us. [*Small chunk of information.*]

CLIENT: Right, I guess I don't know how to relax. I can't drop any of these responsibilities because no one else would do these things. So, I keep pushing and pushing. [*Sustain talk.*]

COACH: You have to take care of your family and all your volunteer jobs, and at the same time, you want to take care of yourself and be healthy. [*Double-sided reflection to build awareness.*]

CLIENT: Yea, that's it. I think it's about time. (*Laughs.*) I'm giving myself some credit for noticing all these symptoms in the first place and taking steps to get help, right? [*Trust is reestablished. Change talk indicates her comfort in considering change.*]

COACH: Absolutely, that's a big first step. [*Affirmation.*] What has you a little baffled is the suggestion that you should cut out some of these things. I get the sense that you feel like folks are asking you to love your people a little less. [*Alignment.*]

CLIENT: That's exactly what it's like! I don't think they understand what they're asking of me. I feel like if I could just hang on until my kids get older and maybe out of school and the community center is up and running, I could relax a little more.

COACH: What might happen when you can relax more? [*Inviting change talk.*]

CLIENT: Hmm. Well, I think first I could focus on my health, maybe get this weight off. Hopefully, I would stop having this racing heart. At least, that's what the doctor thinks. [Shares a story about a recent trip to the Emergency Center for chest pains and rapid heartbeat.] [*Change talk.*] [*Client is more open to what others have said about stress and health.*]

COACH: You might focus on health and your weight. Is there anything else? [*Asking for elaboration and more change talk.*]

CLIENT: And I wouldn't be so irritable at the slightest things with my family. The other day my oldest son was in the car and . . . [Shares a long story about an argument with her son.]	[*Change talk.*] [*Trust.*]
COACH: This isn't like you to be so irritable and argumentative. These things have you thinking it's time to tackle the stress.	[*Affirming, and reflecting change talk.*]
CLIENT: I want to—have to—do something, but it's not so simple. It's not that I'm opposed to reducing stress, but it's impossible to do what they're asking me to do. Truthfully, I know they mean well, and I obviously reached out, so I'm saying, "I need help."	[*Discord with others is softening.*]
COACH: It sounds like you're on board with working on stress management for your health.	[*The coach is waiting for her to state the argument.*]
CLIENT: I think so. You can probably help me with some ideas because you seem to understand where I'm coming from.	[*Partnership.*]
COACH: Yes, and I want to understand more about what you want. What will it be like when you manage your stress?	[*Discord is softened, evoking commitment language.*]
CLIENT: I'm going to feel better. I don't like that awful feeling of being frozen, not able to think about things clearly. The other day I got so angry. [Shares a story about interruptions in her day.] I need to take care of myself, or there won't be enough of me to care for others.	[*Change talk strengthening.*]

This coaching session demonstrates how clients sometimes bring discord into the session and how you can soften it by offering reflections and strategic questions to promote change talk even in these types of circumstances. Notice how the coach listened carefully while the client emptied her basket full of arguments and somewhat narrow thinking. The client seems to have reached her limit of the "you shoulds" from others, so the coach was careful to steer away from the fixing reflex. The MI approach to sustain talk or discord is to temper it because any attempt to refute it will likely make it stronger.

The MI Approach to Discord in a Teaching Example

This example is from a prior job that, in retrospect, demonstrates the beautiful power of MI to guide those who are reluctant to change or those who experience discord with the helpers in their lives. A few years before this incident, I (C. H. L.) shifted my mindset toward my students. Looking back, I now see that I had embraced the MI spirit and methods in my teaching practices, and these became guiding principles for all future interactions in a very satisfying profession.

Joseph was a foot taller and much bigger than his fifth-grade peers. His special education teachers identified him as resistant, rude, and defiant. They warned us teachers to modify expectations and avoid triggering a reactive outburst of defiance, which could become physical.

Since his classroom was across from mine, my students and I often crossed paths with him in the hallway as we transitioned from class to class. Each time we passed, he would press himself up against the wall, slide past us, and keep his eyes laser-focused on the floor. One day a student of mine accidentally bumped him, and Joseph reacted with a yelp and began to yell at the student.

As I approached, Joseph looked down and pushed me out of the way as he lumbered past. My teacher's response was natural, "Joseph, please apologize for that." He reacted with more angry words and gave another hefty shove, which landed me with a thud against the wall. I quickly took my students back to my classroom and asked a substitute to watch them while I went back to talk to Joseph. His teachers were already there, advising me to back away and avoid confrontation. "Just let us handle it." They took him into their classroom and shut the door, but I followed and asked permission to have a private conversation with Joseph in the hallway.

"Joseph, I'm sorry my student bumped you." He persisted in looking down in silence.

"Would you like me to bring him out here to apologize to you?" He shook his head and kept his eyes down. "Joseph, I believe you owe *me* an apology." He was silent and fixed his gaze on the floor. I backed up 3 feet, sensing that I needed to communicate my respect with a physical boundary. He needed his space.

"I can tell you were angry. Would you like to explain what made you so mad?"

He turned his face toward the wall, repeatedly bumping his forehead on the painted concrete block wall. I kept my 3-foot distance and waited for his response.

I remember standing firm, believing he was capable of more and deserved to be heard. I was going to give him a chance to grow, but I knew he had to trust me first. I felt fear, and many "what ifs" began to haunt me. But I would not give up on him.

After waiting what felt like several minutes, I broke the standoff. "Joseph, I believe you have something to say, and what you have to say matters. I have time. I'm listening."

With his forehead propped against the wall, tears began streaming down his cheeks. He began to speak. "No one is nice to me. They do mean things to me and make fun of me and call me stupid and fat. I want to do 'normal' kid stuff at school, and I hate being in that special room away from all the other kids."

The heartbreaking details of his story poured out between his sobs. Keeping my distance, I listened in silence, holding back my own tears.

A shift happened. I saw Joseph in a brand-new way and regretted that I, too, had judged him in the past. But my pity wasn't going to help him. There was a sense of urgency to connect with him and build his confidence, hoping he would become open to learning new skills for managing his behavior. What I was considering was a significant risk but one I chose to take.

"Joseph, I understand how angry that makes you. I'm very sorry you experienced that kind of hurt. Anyone would feel angry like you do."

I mustered the courage to say, "I'm going to turn around and walk to my classroom. I won't pull or force you, but I invite you to follow me. It's your choice to come or not. When we get there, I'll introduce you to my students and ask your teachers if you can stay with us all day." He was silent, but now, he was looking at me. I turned around to face forward and locked my gaze ahead, refusing to glance back to "check" on him, though I could tell he was not walking. I trusted him to make a good choice. It took resolve, but I kept walking forward toward my classroom. As I turned the corner to the room, about 20 feet away from where he stood, I finally heard the slow shuffle of his feet coming toward the classroom. Still looking ahead, I entered the room and told my students we would have a visitor today. About a minute later (which seemed longer), Joseph sheepishly stepped into the room and propped against the doorframe, half out, half in. All the students welcomed him, and a group of boys in the back shouted and waved their hands, "Here, sit next to us; we have room at our table." To my relief and shock, Joseph joined them at the table.

"Guys, why don't you tell our visitor how your group likes to work?" They patiently explained the manners they worked by and demonstrated how to share supplies, wait their turn, respectfully listen to others, and work together on the lessons. After a while, the boy who had accidentally pushed Joseph came up and apologized. We didn't hide our surprise and relief as we witnessed the poignant moment when the boys shook hands.

Joseph stayed all day and asked to come back again the next day. After several days, Joseph's mother called the principal to ask if he could remain in my classroom for the rest of the year. He learned to be pleasant (mostly), social, interactive, and engaged in learning. He got along with his peers and occasionally participated in the typical fifth-grade mischief, always followed by an apology if needed. Whenever his emotions were hard to manage, he followed our plan to go to the back of the room and "refocus," spending time to think, breathe, and choose a new way. His special education teachers were involved, but minimally. After a while, they asked, "What did you do to him? He's so respectful; he's a different kid!"

Looking back, I see the elements of MI at work in this scenario. Joseph's resistance to improve his behavior was, in fact, a deeper issue. He wasn't fighting primarily against school rules or learning objectives but against the students and those of us charged with his care. His reluctance to learn in the face of many obstacles was a normal response, but discord in the relationships with his helpers clouded the path forward and was an impediment to growth. The source of Joseph's defiance, rebellion, reluctance, and anger seemed to be the lack of connection and community with other people.

The goal was to rebuild relationships so we could focus on helping him overcome the learning challenges. If I had pushed and demanded that Joseph come to my room, I'm pretty sure he would have pushed back, internally and maybe even literally. Had I mandated an apology, he might have given one, but it's unlikely he would have joined our classroom and flourished in a community of his peers. With the relationships built, the doorway was flung wide open for Joseph to enter with a new perspective and new possibilities for growth.

Your adult clients may be more subdued in expressing their discord or reluctance to change, but you hear it, nonetheless. A masterful coach learns to recognize discord for what it is and respond accordingly. How you talk and respond to people who are hesitant to change or even those who express discord can shift what you hear from them in return. Discord and sustain talk are not problems with your client but are an opportunity to use your MI skills.

Take It Further

Directions: Read and discuss the questions below with your learning community. Then, for question 3, write an example of the three ways to soften sustain talk and discord.

1. What is the difference between discord and sustain talk? Why is the term "resistance" discouraged when referring to clients?
2. Identify the type of reflections in each of the coach statements below.
   a. You feel this isn't worth your time.
   b. You have absolutely no time to focus on social connections.
   c. You want to be more connected to others, and you haven't found the time.
3. Other than amplified and double-sided reflections, what are three other ways to soften sustain talk and discord? Write examples for each.

Chapter 10

Evoking Hope and Confidence

Hope is believing that the change we desire can be realized and that things will turn out well. Confidence is believing that our attempts to change will result in success. It is possible for clients to be acutely aware of the importance of change and hopeful that life's events will work out positively, but to have little confidence that they can make the needed changes. Evoking hope in coaching may not be necessary when clients have high motivation, clear goals, a sound support system, and robust self-regulation. But with those who struggle to move forward because of failed attempts or difficult circumstances, hope becomes the central focus (Worthen & Isakson, 2010).

Having confidence impacts the activities people attempt, the strength of their efforts, their persistence, and their final success. Clients with high confidence to accomplish a task (self-efficacy) engage more readily, work harder, recover faster from difficulties, and achieve more. The opposite is also true: Clients with low confidence are less likely to commit to taking steps to change (Schunk, 1995).

Using an MI-consistent approach is a way to evoke and strengthen clients' self-efficacy, which in turn influences change. Firming confidence in one's ability to change and doing so in a supportive coach–client relationship plays an essential role in impacting positive behavior (Chariyeva et al., 2013).

FOUR CONSIDERATIONS OF IMPORTANCE AND CONFIDENCE

Refer to Figure 10.1 to decide what might be needed. The first group of people view change as important and feel confident enough to do something

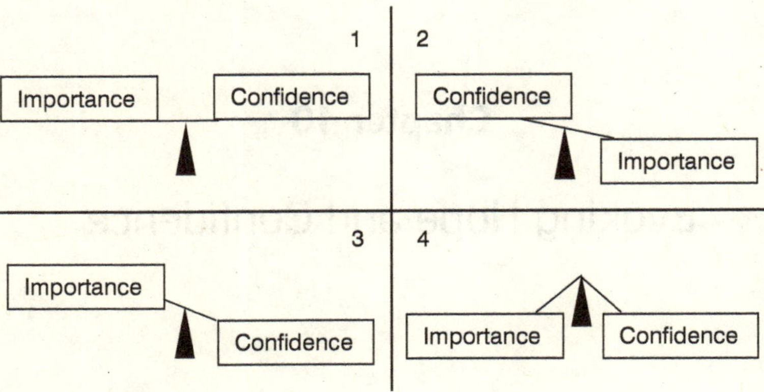

FIGURE 10.1. Importance and confidence.

about it. Those clients may be ready to plan. The second group of people are confident they can change but are not convinced that it's very important. This is where the MI evoking skill begins, and you evoke importance. A third group feels that change is important but lacks the confidence to initiate or sustain action. They may be stuck—temporarily—feeling discouraged or even demoralized by repeated failed attempts. For these people, you focus on evoking confidence. Finally, in quadrant four, you see some people who do not consider a change either important or possible.

WHEN TO EVOKE CONFIDENCE

Often, we see new coaches miss opportunities to evoke change. Perhaps the difficulty arises if you lose sight of where you are, where you are headed, and, most importantly, why. Recall that in engaging, you enter a conversation with clients that fosters the partnership and your working alliance. We like to depict this as a somewhat circular conversation in which you listen, reflect, affirm, summarize, and ask open questions to explore and understand a client's dilemma. You sit with them and empathically listen, something the NBHWC refers to as developing "trust and rapport." You demonstrate accurate empathy and unconditional positive regard, scaffold a way of being with clients, and frame future conversations that honor clients' autonomy, expertise, and ideas for change. Recall that you will don your coaches' CAPE in engaging and all four tasks, working from a rubric of compassion, acceptance, partnership, and empowerment from beginning to end.

But the direction slightly shifts as you enter the focusing task and initiate momentum. The simple diagram in Figure 10.2 is one way to visualize

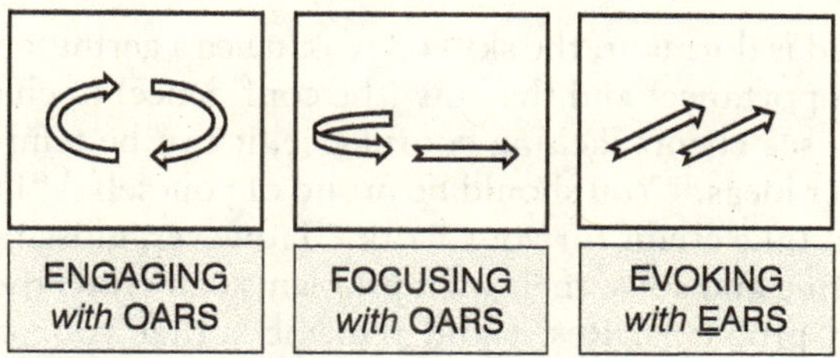

FIGURE 10.2. Flow of MI conversations.

how the conversation implies a forward aim as you search for an agreed-upon destination. In focusing, use the OARS skills while remaining client centered, keeping their agenda and needs foremost as you co-create the target.

Then, as you explore clients' intention–behavior gap and any ambivalence about change, you find that evoking is needed. Where are your clients on the hill of change; do you hear preparatory or mobilizing change talk? How strong is the quality of their motivation, their expressed needs, reasons, and desires to change? Do you detect a consideration of commitment, even in small measures?

Recall that the consideration of motivation is twofold, representing both importance and confidence in the acronym DARN. The "A" refers to a person's perceived ability to make a change, which speaks to confidence. What is the need of the client in front of you? What is their level of importance and confidence? Is the client stalled and hesitant to take action to change? Might this be from discouragement, demoralization, or doubt in their ability? Though you are structuring the conversation to move forward, be cautious not to push ahead prematurely in the presence of low confidence. Self-efficacy is essential to successful change (Bandura, 2000).

In evoking, as Figure 10.2 shows, you adopt a more directional flow in the conversation as you call forth change talk. It's more than the circular nature of engaging or the forward orientation of focusing. You place cones along the road's edge to steer things a particular way, skillfully shifting OARS to EARS, to evoke motivation (Chapter 7). As you turn your attention and energies toward confidence, you are still evoking and looking to find and enlarge upon confidence language. What we said previously about evoking applies here to the vital issue of confidence.

Confidence Talk

When we say clients are "creative, resourceful, and whole," it implies that they already have what they need within themselves. Evoking is searching for and amplifying what exists, not implanting something that is absent.

Though the seed is dormant, the skill of evoking can germinate and nourish the why (the importance) and the how (the confidence) of change.

When you see clients lacking confidence, it can be tempting to try to fix them or offer ideas. "You should be proud of yourself," "I'm thinking of ways you could take credit for your work." However, glossing over clients' attempts to define and solve their own problems can erode their confidence in coping with problems. Resist and remember that your clients are the experts on themselves. Instead, ask open questions that will be answered with confidence talk. Follow up with purposeful reflections that evoke and strengthen confidence language.

The acronym EARS is a way to remember the shift. As we said in Chapter 7, in the evoking task, your open questions become ones that ask for examples, elaboration, and exploration of confidence. This is what we mean by a directional flow. You affirm strengths to lend hope and inspire possibilities. You evoke clients' ideas for change and their confidence in succeeding. You reflect confidence talk and offer summaries about their ability to change.

"What are some ways you think you could do this?"
"If you started tomorrow on this small step, what would you do first?"
"What do you need to happen to make the change successfully?"
"You have many good ideas, and you think your organization skills could help you."
"What gives you the confidence to attempt this?"

You are listening for your clients' expressions of confidence and their ideas for how they might make some changes. As you hear ability language such as *can, could, able to,* and *possible,* you will strengthen that sense of confidence and explore their ideas for how they could succeed.

RESPONDING TO CONFIDENCE TALK

Confidence Ruler

When you ask, "How important is it for you to make this change?" sit back and listen. If clients express high importance, you might also want to know the answer to the second question about confidence, "How confident do you feel about succeeding if you were to decide to make this change?" You could use a scaling question to ask about confidence, "On a scale of 1 to 10, how confident are you to . . . ?" Always follow up with "Why are you not at a (lower number)?" which elicits more confidence talk. Asking the reverse question (about a higher number) will give you sustain talk. Coaching is an authentic, dynamic exchange between you and the client. To avoid becoming formulaic, masterful coaches try to limit the number of these scaling-type questions in a session to no more than two.

Although these two questions provide information for you, their usefulness goes beyond a simple assessment. The rich benefit comes from the follow-up conversation and exploration. Asking these questions is not about gathering data so you can present a plan; it's about evoking your clients' confidence talk and strengthening it when you hear it. As clients listen to themselves making a case for confidence, remember that their own voice has more impact than yours.

What follows is an example of a coaching conversation where the client has high importance and low confidence. This is from a check-in session following a break from 12 weeks of coaching. Notice the use of engaging and evoking skills.

CLIENT: I lost all the good health habits I worked on. I'm sorry, but for some reason, I just stopped doing the things I needed to do. I don't care anymore, and I'm so far down the hole I don't know if I can start back up again.

COACH: You're pretty discouraged today. What do you need to start caring again?

CLIENT: That's a good question. I almost didn't show up today, but I thought you might be able to help. Do you have any ideas for me?

COACH: Sure, we can talk about a few things to try, but first, since you know yourself best, what are some ideas you have for moving up out of the hole? [*Emphasizing autonomy.*]

CLIENT: Hmm, I know this is important and how much it helped me, but I guess I don't care enough to start doing anything. If I did, I would probably have done it.

COACH: It's important, but you're not sure you can do it. [*Reflecting low confidence.*]

CLIENT: Yeah, that's it! I'm not even sure I could do it if I tried.

COACH: You said it helped you. What were some of the benefits you felt when you took better care of your health? [*Evoking.*]

CLIENT: I lost weight, my blood pressure was lower, my cholesterol numbers were good, and I felt much better in my body. I had more confidence, too.

COACH: You liked having that confidence. How do you feel now? [*Reflecting meaning, evoking.*]

CLIENT: Gosh, I feel pretty sad, and I'm not happy about myself. I'm happily married, and life is good in many ways, but I don't like living this way. I'm overweight, my back hurts again, and my blood pressure is up. I feel horrible.

COACH: You love feeling healthy, but you're not the "healthy you" that you believe is best; that is the real you. [*Reflecting ambivalence.*]

CLIENT: (*in tears*) You're right; I know it's not me, not the *real* me, or the self with a capital "S," as you've said. Right now, I have to focus on loving so many other people in my life, like my family, houseguests, and my patients. We're moving to a new house next week, and there isn't time to care for me. You have to love and care about yourself first to be able to love others. Because if you have it, you can give it. [*Reasons to change, making pro arguments to self.*]

COACH: I see how sad this makes you. Loving yourself is your way of loving others from a generous place. What would it take to love yourself first again? [*Empathic reflection, evoking ability.*]

CLIENT: I know what to do; I'm just stuck. You can give love, but if it's not from a good place, it's unhealthy and not balanced. I put loving others above loving myself, but I don't know why. I'm a doer for others, but I need to be a doer for myself. Then, I can probably be a better person for others. [*Ability language.*]

COACH: You want to be better for yourself and others. On a scale of 1 to 10, if 10 is very confident and 1 is not very confident, how confident are you that you could restart some self-care habits? [*Confidence ruler evoking question.*]

CLIENT: I might be a 3.

COACH: Okay, you're at a 3. Why aren't you at 1? [*Evoking confidence.*]

CLIENT: (*Laughs.*) Ha! When I came in here today, I was at a zero! I guess I'm at a 3 now because I know what it's like to feel good about myself. I already did this once this year, and it felt great.

COACH: What else?

CLIENT: I was able to smile and not fake it. I was really happy and not so damn worried about bending down and feeling back pain or getting out of breath to walk up the stairs and not being embarrassed about my weight. I remember how good that felt!

COACH: It sounds like you can imagine it right now, just talking it out, and you want that back again. [*Reflecting confidence and hope.*]

CLIENT: I can! It's a great feeling; once you know it, you know what you're missing when it's gone. This sounds silly, but I forgot about all that for a while. Talking about it out loud right now, it seems pretty straightforward. But I'm convinced I can do this because I've done it before. I *can* do this. [*Confidence language.*]

COACH: What would be a good, small first step to get started again? [*Evoking, emphasizing autonomy.*]

Finding and Affirming Strengths

When self-confidence is low and hope is diminished, there are ways to help your client. Acknowledging what is "right" about people and what unique strengths they possess goes a long way to bolster confidence and self-worth. Begin a search for your clients' inner resources and strengths that could be helpful in their current struggles. You can ask questions that directly target your clients' positive traits and character strengths. Some coaches like to start by having clients take a simple character strengths survey and then follow up with reflective listening to explore further (see Chapter 5).

Another, more structured activity is to use a list of 100 positive adjectives, shown in Table 10.1 (Miller & Rollnick, 2013). Say to clients, "Take a look at this list of strengths that people have and circle at least five that describe you best." Once again, the value of these activities is in the MI style of open questions and reflective listening that follow. You evoke the process of self-discovery and ask clients to dig deep and uncover the strengths, qualities, and skills they already possess.

While serving as an instructional coach for teachers, I (C. H. L.) used to caution, "Don't crack the egg." Usurping students' discovery process could weaken their learning and, most importantly, their developing self-confidence. MI methods follow a similar purpose by allowing people to speak about how and why change could happen and what they might do to

TABLE 10.1. Some Characteristics of Successful Changers

Accepting	Committed	Flexible	Persevering	Stubborn
Active	Competent	Focused	Persistent	Thankful
Adaptable	Concerned	Forgiving	Positive	Thorough
Adventuresome	Confident	Forward-looking	Powerful	Thoughtful
Affectionate	Considerate	Free	Prayerful	Tough
Affirmative	Courageous	Happy	Quick	Trusting
Alert	Creative	Healthy	Reasonable	Trustworthy
Alive	Decisive	Hopeful	Receptive	Truthful
Ambitious	Dedicated	Imaginative	Relaxed	Understanding
Anchored	Determined	Ingenious	Reliable	Unique
Assertive	Die-hard	Intelligent	Resourceful	Unstoppable
Assured	Diligent	Knowledgeable	Responsible	Vigorous
Attentive	Doer	Loving	Sensible	Visionary
Bold	Eager	Mature	Skillful	Whole
Brave	Earnest	Open	Solid	Willing
Bright	Effective	Optimistic	Spiritual	Winning
Capable	Energetic	Orderly	Stable	Wise
Careful	Experienced	Organized	Steady	Worthy
Cheerful	Faithful	Patient	Straight	Zealous
Clever	Fearless	Perceptive	Strong	Zestful

Note. From Miller (2004). In the public domain.

succeed. The power lies in people (re)discovering and articulating their own arguments for confidence about change. Coaching is less about your skill at spotting strengths and more about you handing the magnifying glass over to your clients.

Recalling Past Learnings and Successes

In addition to evoking strengths, you can boost confidence by asking clients to remember past experiences when they tried something that seemed hard to do but they succeeded. Masterful coaches use MI to expand the conversation beyond a collective list. Use EARS to explore in more depth, asking for examples and details about what strategies they used and how they prepared and persevered through to succeed. What learning and insight did they gain in that situation that they can apply now? What did they do to get started? What obstacles got in the way, and how did they navigate through them? Help them overlay these specific strategies, learnings, and skills and apply them in a broader way in the present circumstance. In this rich conversation, you could also ask clients to explore other positive resources and supports that might be available to help.

Reframing

When things go wrong, humans want to find a cause for it. If people feel at fault, this can give rise to negative feelings, which may generate low confidence and even hopelessness. On the other hand, if people feel that something unstable such as external factors or unfavorable conditions are at play, they can maintain hope for the future. External factors might include effort or luck, "This wasn't my time," or "I can do it when I give more effort." Therefore, helping clients reframe thoughts of personal failure can circumvent the negative emotional consequences and the resulting behaviors. Based on abundant research, cause stimulates emotions, which in turn spur action (Weiner, 2018).

Help clients reframe and reinterpret failures as attempts or "tries" that demonstrate their commitment, determination, or fierce tenacity. Encourage them to view change as a spiral rather than a linear path. Prochaska's depiction of an upward spiral gives perspective, helping clients understand that most changers cycle through three or four attempts before making it to the successful exit of the cycle (see Figure 10.3).

Although some people can change with no false starts or lapses, that is rare. Prochaska's research followed changers for 2 years and found that only 5% went through without even one setback (1994). Offer your clients the perspective that a misstep does not mean all is lost and that failures can be opportunities for feedback. These experiences can be seen as recycling, not relapsing, on an upward journey of growth and discovery. A few

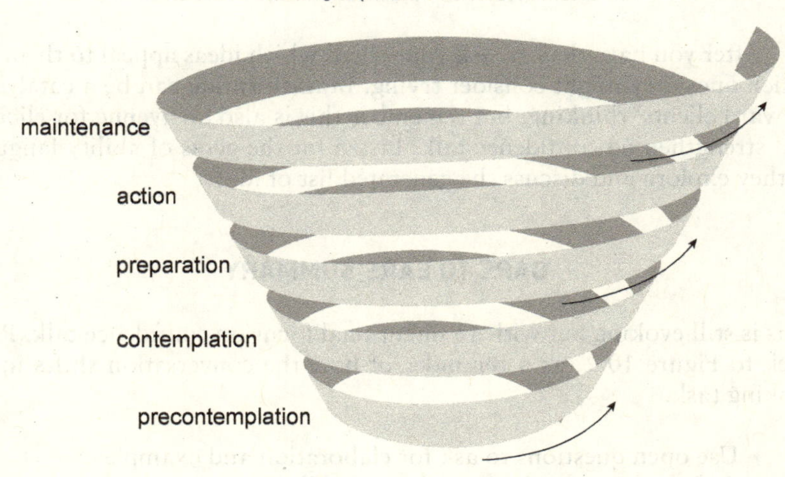

FIGURE 10.3. The spiral of change. Based on Prochaska et al. (1994).

setbacks tend to make people feel like they are going in circles. While you can acknowledge and demonstrate compassion for your clients, help them reframe and see that the circles are spiraling upward toward the exit point. Help clients abandon the idea that they need to return to square one and start all over. You can influence the surge of hopefulness and confidence by using reframing to evoke confidence.

Reframing mindset is often a primary focus in coaching. You help clients hurdle the obstacles that get in the way of change, especially those clients who feel stuck in doubt, delay, and discouragement and have low confidence in making the changes they want. The antidote is to help clients surface their beliefs, find alternatives, and identify actions to take that grow from these beliefs. (See Handout 10.1, "Learned Optimism," online at *www.guilford.com/lanier-materials*, for more on helping clients develop an optimistic versus pessimistic perspective.)

Brainstorming

Clients are indeed creative, but creativity can become clouded by a loss of hope and confidence. Brainstorming is a way to jump-start the problem-solving process. Use this strategy when clients ask for ideas or when they seem stuck and unable to find possibilities. Start by asking for a steady flow of all ideas, no matter how unrealistic or silly they may seem. Ideas are not up for critique, so gather them briefly in pursuit of a range of options. It's fine to offer some of your ideas, but this activity is a way to stimulate a client's divergent thinking.

After you have the list, ask your client which ideas appeal to them and which ones they might consider trying. Brainstorming can be a catalyst to forward clients' thinking, but remember this is also an avenue for eliciting and strengthening confidence talk. Listen for the gems of ability language as they explore and discuss the generated list of ideas.

OARS TO EARS SUMMARY

This is still evoking but with an intentional focus on confidence talk. Refer back to Figure 10.2, as a reminder of how the conversation shifts in the evoking task.

- Use open questions to ask for elaboration and examples.
- Affirm the person's strengths and abilities.
- Reflect the person's self-confidence language.
- Summarize the person's reasons that change is possible.

Coaching with EARS is not a matter of finding the magic bullet to build confidence: It's about sitting with clients and allowing them to process their doubts and timidity about change. The skill of reflection remains key as you become a compassionate witness, listening deeply for and reflecting on clients' thoughts, beliefs, and perceptions about their ability to change.

Get comfortable with silence and long pauses, allowing time for clients to examine lessons from failed attempts. Guide them to reframe experiences and build capacity for success, supporting them to find a new perspective beyond one that is eclipsed by current doubt and delay. Foster a feeling of being supported as they search for the courage to try again.

Often, the process of building engagement is medicine itself: "A supportive other can help mobilize hope and renewed effort" (Bohart & Tallman, 2010). People rarely have this kind of relationship with someone who would help them process their struggles. Certainly, you help them consider other resources for support, but remember that the coach–client relationship is an excellent place to start.

Coaching Sample: Strengthening Confidence

This is a case where the client struggled with confidence.

CLIENT: It *could* happen, but I'm not confident it'll happen this weekend. I haven't made it 3 weeks without drinking alcohol in a while. This	[*Low confidence*.]

weekend will be 3 weeks, and I don't know if I can do it.

COACH: It's hard for you to resist, but you want a change; you want to kick that habit. [*Reflecting ambivalence, ending with change talk.*]

CLIENT: I really do. That's the part I don't get. I can work out at the gym 4 or 5 days a week and work a full-time job, but I can't stop myself from eating a large pizza and drinking, especially when my wife's gone. I can't explain it.

COACH: You're successful at plenty of things. [*Affirm strengths.*]

CLIENT: Thanks, I really forget that sometimes. It's like two people are living my life. I'm a responsible software engineer by day but act like a college kid at night. *(Laughs.)* My wife gave me an ultimatum; either get my weight under control and stop drinking, or there will be trouble.

My doctor told me I was at high risk for disease if I didn't lose weight. I guess the two things go together, you know when you drink, you have to eat more, at least that's what I do. I make a no-excuses decision at first, and after a few drinks, I just give in and eat whatever I want. There are lots of other things I want to do, but I have a few drinks, and all those goals disappear. Let's talk about the drinking and save the food discussion for next time. I really want to change and be free of this craziness. [*Desire, reasons, needs.*]

COACH: It's urgent. [*Slight amplified reflection.*]

CLIENT: It is. I've tried lots of times to quit drinking, but like I said, I haven't made it past 3 weeks yet, and if you can get past 3 weeks, you've broken a habit. Is that right?

COACH: Sure, it depends on how long you've had the habit, but generally, it can take 2 to 3 weeks to get past the most [*Offer information, evoking possibilities.*]

challenging part. What will it be like to get past this?

CLIENT: Well, I want to keep my marriage and my job, and not get sick, so I'm hoping this is it, that I can do it.

COACH: Job stability and a good marriage. So, what's your plan for this weekend? [*Reflection, followed by evoking question.*]

CLIENT: It was easier the last 2 weeks because I was busy, but the real test will be this weekend because I'll be home alone. That's where I need your help.

COACH: You need a plan. [*Reflecting, not solving.*]

CLIENT: Yep, if my wife wasn't leaving for the weekend, it might not be so hard. I'm not confident it's going to happen. [*Low confidence.*]

COACH: You mentioned going to the gym and working out. You're able to do what most people would consider hard. What do you know about yourself that helps you get to the gym and do your workouts? [*Reframe, affirm, and open question to evoke strengths.*]

CLIENT: Yeah, I mean, nothing comes before my workout time. It's crazy, but I love it. I might be the heaviest person using weights at the gym. And lately, I've joined an indoor cycling group, and we have races with other teams remotely. To answer your question, I'm stubborn and determined.

COACH: How does determination help with your gym commitment? [*Evoking confidence.*]

CLIENT: I don't like to let people down. If I commit to a race, then I'm going to show up. For the past 2 weeks, I didn't drink on Friday night because I knew I was going to race on Saturday morning, and I didn't want to let my team down. Other people depended on me.

COACH: You have the drive and personal integrity. [*Affirming strengths.*]

CLIENT: Yeah, I guess so. (*Long pause.*)

COACH: Give an example of the last time you used integrity. [*Evoking positive traits.*]

CLIENT: Well, every day, I've shown up at the gym, not just Saturday.

COACH: What got you to the gym on those other days when you're not part of a team race? [*Evoking question to explore strengths.*]

CLIENT: That's easy; I committed to *myself!* Last Saturday, I had a stiff back, but I went anyway and walked on the treadmill going really slow for 30 minutes. I haven't been able to walk any distance when my back's tight like that. So, I was saying, "Well, I guess I'll never hike again." I got out of bed, stretched a little, and went straight to the gym. I walked 30 minutes at a 3% incline at 2.5 miles an hour. And yeah, my back was fine. So that was uplifting and proved that I *can* do it. I just need to work on it. That was probably the biggest breakthrough. I know I can cycle and do non-weight-bearing exercises when my back is so bad. Carrying all this weight, it's hard, and moving with all that, that's what's in question for me. [*Ability language.*] [*Client builds a case for confidence.*]

COACH: I see what you mean about stubbornness! That integrity said, "I'm going to do something right for me." [*Affirm strengths.*]

CLIENT: And I did it without my wife! That wasn't for anybody else's benefit but my own. [Confidence *growing.*]

COACH: What's the importance of doing it without her? [*Evoking, elaboration.*]

CLIENT: I think doing it on my own, it's for me, not just going along with what she says or does. It's doing something extra, maybe something extra and different, only for me.

COACH: When you do things for yourself, you get a different result than doing it for someone else. [*Reflecting discrepancy.*]

CLIENT: That's difficult because I don't often do things for myself. I'll do them like when I'm cycling, and we're all one crew. We're all on the same team, so the miles I cycle count for everyone. So, I keep cycling for everyone else, not for me. But we have a coach who always asks, "What's your why? What are you doing for yourself today?" So that makes you refocus and think about it, but I don't know, I want to stick to the plan this weekend, mostly for myself. And to prove that I can do something for myself; I don't do that a lot. It's hard to answer. [*Low confidence. His reflections indicate a mindset shift.*]

COACH: Earlier, you mentioned that you'd steered away from the croissants and sweets at the office. What do you think was pulling you to make that choice? [*Linking reflection. Evoking, exploring broader strengths.*]

CLIENT: I think I'm trying to have a little more self-compassion and self-care. [*Possibility thinking, confidence talk.*]

COACH: Self-compassion helped you choose to avoid sweets. What would self-compassion look like this weekend? [*Reflection and open evoking question.*]

CLIENT: Hmm, that's the hard part. Avoiding sweets is one thing but getting past 3 weeks without alcohol is the hard part for me. The tricky part will be Saturday late afternoon after cycling for the day and then going home to do chores. I'm stuck, and really, I don't know.

COACH: Okay, let's brainstorm. You mentioned creativity was one of your signature strengths, so how about throwing out some creative ideas, even the ones that seem unrealistic at first? We're looking for a stream of ideas, as many as we can think of. How does that sound? [*Inviting brainstorming.*]

CLIENT: Yeah, I'm good at divergent thinking; remember, I'm a software engineer. (*Smiling.*)

COACH: Okay, how could you use self-compassion to avoid alcohol this weekend and get past the 3-week mark? [*Connect strengths to the current situation.*]

CLIENT: I could lock myself in my car! (*Jokingly.*)

COACH: (*Laughs.*) Okay, what else?

CLIENT: Speaking of creativity, I could get my sketch pad and paints out and start designing something, maybe a vision board. [*Awareness of strengths, opening up to possibilities.*]

COACH: That actually sounds fun! What else? [*Evoking.*]

CLIENT: I could invite a buddy over. But wait, I don't want anyone with me because most of my friends are drinking buddies. I could just pull out that journal we talked about.

COACH: Writing down your thoughts would help. What kinds of things would you write? [*Evoking examples.*]

CLIENT: Remember last week when we talked about how I was grieving over losing alcohol and bad food? I said they were bad friends, and they had to go.

COACH: Yes, I remember. We said you wanted to "break up" with your bad lovers. [*Linking summary.*]

CLIENT: Maybe I could write a letter to alcohol and break up officially. Like, write down what it brings and takes away from me. I could make it fun. I might use my sketch pad to draw out what that might look like, and make that my vision board. [*Energy shift around creativity and possibility.*]

COACH: You're excited about it, and this idea resonates with you. How do you feel after creating this list? [*Acknowledge and reflect emotions.*]

CLIENT: Well, it's easier said than done, isn't it? But I think I could do the letter and vision board. You wouldn't believe some of the complicated software I've designed. You have to be good at problem solving in my field.

COACH: Your problem-solving skills help you do complex things. You're stubborn and determined, and you have personal integrity. [*A collecting summary of strengths.*]

CLIENT: Um, I'm probably stronger than I'm feeling right now and stronger than I've given myself credit for. Because despite being a little bit down and not sleeping well last night, I still stuck to it today and did what I had to, I mean, what I *wanted* to do. Not what I was *supposed* to do, but what I *wanted* to do. [*Mindset shifts. Confidence talk is stronger.*]

COACH: You're doing it for yourself, not others. [*Reflecting meaning.*]

CLIENT: Yeah, and I think trying not to live in the negative, like you said, rather than coming to the third week with a sense of dread, I approach it with curiosity. So, it's been a different approach for me this week because I normally would have quit by now.

COACH: What kinds of thoughts are you having about this weekend? [*Open question to explore.*]

CLIENT: Yeah, it's harder with my wife not here, but I told myself I wasn't going to drink, and sometimes that's not good enough. It's tough. I had a major trigger last week when some buddies had me over.

COACH: You're doing it, but it is one of the hardest things you've ever done. What did you say to get past it? [*Choosing to reflect change talk, evoking past strategies.*]

CLIENT: Well, I'm not having any alcohol; that's all there is to it. It's not an option, and it wasn't an option when my wife was in the house. I have a bottle of bourbon, and I could have already opened it, but it's just not an option. I could have already opened it, but I'm not going to. That's what I have to keep in mind. It's not something I do. [*Strong confidence and commitment talk.*]

This client entered the session with high importance and low confidence. In a brief coaching conversation, he gained confidence, strengthened his resolve, and committed to a feasible plan for a no-alcohol weekend. The coach resisted the fixing reflex but instead spent time reflecting and calling forth confidence by reviewing the broad scope of the client's capabilities and characteristics. The client followed up on Monday with this personal text message: "I made it to 26 days! I did it!"

Take It Further

Directions: Work in your learning community to discuss and answer the questions below. Handouts 10.1–10.4 are available at *www.guilford.com/lanier-materials*.

1. Review the strategies for evoking confidence in Table 10.2 (on p. 194). Read the strategies in Column A, then answer the prompts in Column B. Some questions challenge you to consider not only the "what" but also the "why" and "how" of these strategies.
2. Read Handout 10.1, "Learned Optimism." Then, discuss with a partner what MI strategies you would use with a client who tends toward pessimism.
3. Read Handout 10.2, "Applying the Strategies." Work with a partner to write an appropriate reflection or question in the engaging, focusing, or evoking tasks.
4. Read Handout 10.3, "Being a Compassionate Witness." Reflect on the "do this!" and "avoid that!" lists, then share with a partner which of the items on the list are your strengths and which ones you would like to focus on for growth.
5. Bonus: Read Handout 10.4, "An Example of the Power of Evoking in Young Children." Can you describe how you have used evoking in either coaching or another situation?

TABLE 10.2. Challenge Your Thinking: Evoking Confidence

A: Strategies to evoke confidence	B: Prompts to consider the best ways to use the strategies
Open questions	How do open questions shift in the evoking process?
Lend hope, inspire possibilities	A client says, "I don't know if I can." What would you say?
Find strengths	What might result from the coach overusing "strength spotting"?
Affirm strengths	Which methods might you use to affirm strengths?
Reflect confidence talk	Why would you reflect confidence talk? Give an example.
Scaling questions (1–10)	What is the follow-up question and why is it the most important question?
Recall past learning and success	Why ask the client to look beyond the current change target?
Reframing	How would you help a client reframe the statement "I have no willpower"?
Brainstorming	What might happen if you (the coach) offer a lot of ideas in a brainstorming activity?

Chapter 11

Coaching with Neutrality

Coaching someone toward their desired change is always done with equanimity. As you advocate to support clients toward *their* chosen goals, you never usurp their autonomy by inserting your agenda over theirs. However, if a client asks for help to stop smoking or regain their health by choosing better foods, you are certainly there to support them in achieving their goals. You use powerful questioning to forward the momentum toward growth, all within MI-consistent methods. Here, we consider those times when you pull back and intentionally refrain from being directional, deciding instead to remain neutral.

A distinctive component of MI is the directional evoking described in Chapter 7. Coaching with neutrality adopts the assumption that you can influence an ambivalent person's choice; research has shown that coaches can influence their clients (Cialdini, 2007). For this reason, your choice to remain neutral is an intention to *not* influence the decision in one direction or the other.

How do you decide when to coach with neutrality or use directional evoking? There are no hard rules for this, but we encourage you to filter your decision through both your personal and professional ethics and your set of values when deciding to influence or not. Your intuition and judgment and your experiences will also sway the decision. We hope that as you learn the skill of remaining neutral, you pay attention to how you can be directional when you choose to be.

One apparent reason to coach your clients toward a particular choice is that they have asked you to do so. If your moral conscience is at ease, and you have no ethical lines to cross, you ally with your clients on the agreed-upon goal. In all these situations, the essential first step is wearing your CAPE and engaging and ensuring that clients feel safe and empowered to explore all the possibilities.

In the focusing task, you may become aware of specific issues that do not warrant leaning toward one choice or the other. The issue is not can you but *should* you influence your client in a particular direction. Without any clear legal or ethical considerations at play, you may decide that it's inappropriate to favor one choice over another, and so you choose to refrain from influencing your client.

If you choose *not* to evoke in one direction, are you still using MI? As we have said, the intent of MI is to evoke the client's own arguments and motivations for change, typically with the goal of steering toward a specific outcome. Coaching with neutrality allows your clients to choose among difficult choices—with your assistance—without your influence either way. If clients progress beyond an uncomfortable, stuck place and either make a decision or at least begin the decision-making process, we consider this to be successful coaching, no matter what you call it.

DECIDING WHEN TO COACH WITH NEUTRALITY

Is it ethical to influence a person to choose one thing over another? An early criticism of MI was that it was a gentle way to manipulate people to do something they may not otherwise want. In the third edition of *Motivational Interviewing: Helping People Change,* Miller and Rollnick (2013) answered this by introducing the component of compassion, which serves as your guide when considering these ethical questions. Compassion is not a set of skills to master, but is an intention permeating everything you do in coaching. When considering whether to coach with neutrality, anchor the question with a compassionate interest in the person's well-being and let it steer you to either stay neutral or become directional.

Some cases fall into a gray zone, where you feel it would be ethically wrong to sway the client either way. You may have an opinion but believe the choice rests solely with your client, so it feels appropriate to remain neutral. It is in these untidy spaces in the middle where you must pay attention to your heart and find clarity.

Neutrality with Referring Practitioners, Sponsors, or Third Parties

At times, in health coaching, you may see clients as part of a collaborative care team where practitioners prescribe and then send their patients for coaching related to a specific goal. For example, clients have a directive for medication, supplementation, diet, or related lifestyle changes. In these cases, there is an implied, built-in directional change goal. But suppose clients are ambivalent about the prescription and, for example, choose to forgo the medication for a more holistic approach. How would you coach these clients? Who are you responsible to in these cases? Or consider the client who wants to take medication to control diabetes instead of making dietary changes, "Because I want to keep eating the way I like." Would you remain neutral in this case? While there are ethical and professional standards for coaching, we strongly encourage you to connect with supervisors, mentors, and other coaches for ongoing dialogue to explore these questions. (See the ICF Code of Ethics online at *www.guilford.com/lanier-materials*.) Regardless, coaching with MI will ensure that you remain in a place of compassion and choose what is in the best interest of your clients. We are not offering a simple formula to determine when to evoke and when to remain neutral. As we said, the answers are informed by your personal and professional ethics. Then, sometimes, the decision to stay neutral is made in the context of a team approach among you, the referring practitioner, and the client. (See the "Take It Further" section at the end of the chapter for more discussion of this decision process.) Sometimes, without an opinion or a mandate, you may want to provide information to help clients make an informed decision, and you refrain from influencing their decision beyond that.

Cases When Neutrality Is Considered

As mentioned, most scenarios fall into two general categories: first, when you want to use directional evoking, and second, when there is an absence of clear guidelines or any legal or professional obligations and you choose to remain neutral. Consider these cases below and decide if you could (or could not) remain neutral. Do you have strong reactions or opinions to some of these? Be tuned in to any inclination to sway the decision one way based on what you believe is morally or ethically right. How would you coach these clients?

1. A 19-year-old is deciding between going to college or starting a job as a yoga instructor.
2. An engineer wants to know if she should stay with a high-pressure, high-paying job or choose a start-up company with less pay but opportunities for creative design.
3. A woman contemplates divorcing her husband of 25 years for a new lover.
4. A patient decides whether to forgo traditional cancer treatment in favor of holistic approaches.
5. A 54-year-old dentist is at a crossroads, wondering if he should leave his practice (where he has lost his passion) and choose a new vocation, which would upset his wife.

6. A woman wonders if she should quit her job to care for her parent at home or hire someone to do that.
7. A mother disagrees with her husband and wants to take her 16-year-old daughter for an abortion.
8. A man wonders if he should become a vegetarian to reach his goal of losing weight and feeling more energetic.

Informing Clients about Neutrality

If you choose neutrality, the best approach is to be transparent. Remember that clients who are stuck are most likely in a great deal of discomfort, and it's normal for them to look to their coach for direction. Be alert for clients to experience even more discomfort when you inform them of your intention to stay neutral. Here are a few ways to support your client:

- Express your desire to help them explore their dilemma.
- Be transparent and tell them your intention to remain neutral.
- Explain that your goal is to help them decide and move forward however they choose.
- Empathize with them and normalize the discomfort of feeling stuck as a natural consequence of making difficult choices.
- Coach toward building capacity, developing confidence, and exploring possibilities.

Strategies for Coaching with Neutrality

When you decide it's necessary and appropriate to advocate neutrality, MI offers guidance about how *not* to steer your clients in a particular direction. First, recall the multiple research findings on MI that confirm the power of evoking, of using your words to raise the likelihood of change talk and change. Neutrality, then, would involve an intentional response so that you would *not* sway the decision either way, even inadvertently.

Decisional Balance Tool

Recall that in Chapter 7, we asked you to consider whether or not to use the decisional balance tool with ambivalent clients who are in the contemplation stage of change since equally voicing pros and cons often results in no change (Magill et al., 2013). Using the tool would evoke both sustain talk and change talk, which can result in maintaining ambivalence and a *decreased* commitment to change (Miller & Rose, 2015). If your primary aim is *not* to steer the conversation one way but to help the client to grapple with all the pros and cons of a decision, the decisional balance tool is a practical resource. See Figure 11.1 for a completed decisional balance tool (and a blank Handout 11.1 online at *www.guilford.com/lanier-materials*).

Allow clients time to explore the four boxes in the decisional balance tool. If more responses are stacked in boxes 1 and 4 (pros of change and cons of not changing), then change is likely to happen. If responses in boxes 2 and 3 (cons of change and pros of no change) outweigh those in boxes 1 and 4, change is less likely to happen. Ambivalence sounds like equal arguments for each of the four squares.

Benefits/Pros of making a change 1	**Benefits/Pros of not making a change** 2
(Pros of leaving the current relationship) • *I wouldn't be anxious about a future with someone who's so different than me.* • *I could start searching for a better partner.* • *I'd have more time to work on my relationships with family and friends.* • *I might find a partner who shares my goals and encourages me to keep growing.* • *I could get back to being more positive and happy.*	*(Pros of staying in the current relationship)* • *He can be supportive at times.* • *He provides some companionship.* • *I wouldn't have to enter the dating scene again.*
Costs/Cons of making a change 3	**Costs/Cons of not changing** 4
(Cons of leaving the current relationship) • *I've invested a lot of time into this.* • *I don't want to start dating again.* • *I might lose the support I have now and feel sad for a while.*	*(Cons of staying in the relationship)* • *I might not be at peace if I stayed.* • *We don't share similar values in life.* • *I wouldn't be able to work on my personal growth goals as much as I'd like.* • *I'd miss out on social activities and being with friends because he prefers to stay home.* • *I might not find a better partner.*

FIGURE 11.1. Example of a completed decisional balance tool.

Remember that if you chose to practice directional evoking, you would pay attention to squares 1 and 4 (change talk). You would not ignore the other boxes but you would focus energy and coach conversations around the responses in favor of change. The original purpose of the decisional balance tool is to give all boxes equal consideration, and this can help clients feel satisfied that they considered all the possibilities they were aware of at the time.

If your clients find it cumbersome to complete the 4-box form, you can offer a simple 2-column pros-versus-cons format. Another option is to have a conversation and ask clients to explore their pros and cons verbally. Afterward, they can write these down in the form if they choose.

Coaching Sample: Coaching with Neutrality

Below is a portion of a coaching session with a young woman deciding whether to stay at a job or go home to pursue college or another career path.

COACH: Hi, Katelyn. Your mother referred you to me because you're making some important and challenging decisions about college or your current job.

KATELYN: Yeah, I want to decide whether to stay here at this job or go home and start college, and because I'm so wishy-washy, I have panic attacks a lot, and I'm unhappy. I knew what I wanted, but after starting this new job, which was my dream job, I miss home and wonder if I made the wrong choice. [*Choosing between options.*]

COACH: This is an important decision, and you want to do the right thing. That must be hard to be at your dream job and feel so unsure. [*Empathy.*]

KATELYN: Yeah, thanks; it's hard, and no one else understands my problem because it appears I got my wish, but now I only complain. I'm independent, and I don't want to burden anyone else with this. Usually, I know when to walk away; I'm not a quitter. But if I leave this job, I need to know what to do next. That's what I hope you can do; show me the best decision. I feel stuck.

COACH: You're feeling unhappy, and I understand that. In fact, Katelyn, that's normal for people feeling stuck between hard decisions. We can explore this issue as we go along. But instead of telling you which decision to make, it's best for you if I stay neutral so you can consider all your options. How does that sound to you?

[*Inform, empathize, and normalize emotions.*]

KATELYN: That's probably best. I'm not clear right now, but I know being here at this job, I'm missing my family and being in the "flow" the way I like. The surroundings here are not warm and artistic, not inspiring at all. It'll be good to talk about this with someone.

COACH: Before we start, what do you think is a good outcome for our work today?

[*Open question, honor autonomy, partnership.*]

KATELYN: It'd be good if I could just talk about the options. We used a pros-versus-cons list in our persuasive writing class. Maybe I need one of those.

COACH: Would it be ok to explore what's most important to you first, because that could make the pros-versus-cons list a bit more clear? (*Katelyn agrees.*) A minute ago, you mentioned things like independence and finishing things. What else do you know about yourself; what things are most important to you?

[*Open questions to explore core values.*]

KATELYN: I have the "most important" values list from last week. The top five are passion, family, autonomy, self-knowledge, and industry. (*Laughs.*) I'm laughing because passion is definitely me. I have to be "in the flow," or I'm not happy. I exercise, run, do yoga, create art, and write. And self-knowledge is *so* true because I'm an observer of other people. I sit back and analyze why someone says something or what they're thinking. I can tell when someone isn't

[*Clarifying values can help with the focusing task.*]

genuine; they're putting on a show. Actually, I analyze myself like that, too, which is why I chose self-knowledge.

COACH: So, passion, being in the "flow," and you're good at self-knowledge, and spotting when something is genuine. What else on that list feels important to mention? [*Summary, affirmations.*]

KATELYN: I think industry is about not wanting to be a slacker and finishing hard things. I've pushed past some tough stuff before. (*Long pause*) Maybe that's why it's hard to leave my job.

COACH: You're certainly industrious, and that quality has helped you in the past. But you think it also might keep you from leaving. Ok, how do you feel about starting the pros-versus-cons list now? [*Affirming, reflecting both sides to avoid influencing.*]

KATELYN: Yea, I agree. As we've talked, I've already seen some advantages of leaving.

COACH: Here's a form that other clients like to use. Take a look and see if this would be helpful for you. (*Katelyn agrees.*) [*Decisional balance tool.*]

KATELYN: So, in box 1, do I list the pros of leaving the job, starting college, or coming home and starting another career?

COACH: We could do it that way, or we can make a different pros list for each thing you mentioned: leaving the job, starting college, or getting another job. What do you think you'd like to do? [*Partnership, and honoring autonomy.*]

KATELYN: I want to talk about the pros and cons of leaving that job.

COACH: Once you're satisfied that you thought of everything for each box, we can discuss it. [Explains the tool, gives time to finish.]

KATELYN: Here are my lists for boxes 1 and 4. The pros of leaving the job are that I would be with my family and be around authentic people. I'd see them and enjoy the weather changes. I'd probably have time for my art and being in the flow. The cons of not leaving are I may become more and more unhappy. I might neglect self-care, which is important to me. It's hard to get in the flow when I'm here, and it's just not an inspiring place.

COACH: Okay, what about boxes 2 and 3? (*Gives equal attention to each box.*)

KATELYN: For box 2, the pros of staying, I like my roommates, and they can be helpful, like when I had a fender bender the other day. Also, I want this job on my resume, and I guess this experience is helping me learn something.
And for box 3, the cons of leaving are that I wouldn't have this on my resume, and I'd be scared to go home and not know what to do next, like a job or starting college.

COACH: Okay, you'd be with your family and other authentic people and do art and more "flow" activities. But if you stayed, you might be more unhappy, and wouldn't do "flow" activities because you're not inspired. For box 2, the pros of staying there, you'd add this job on your resume, have roommates, and you could learn something.

For box 3, the cons of leaving, you wouldn't have this job on your resume, and you might not know what to do once you got home. Is there anything else?

[*Summarize to include material from all four boxes equally.*]

KATELYN: Now that I hear what I said, I think this is beginning to put things in perspective. Diving into my values felt kind of centering because I sometimes feel very lost. So, having that kind of rock to go back to is good. It's like we were trying to figure out *me* and not so much about "what I'm doing." This helped me get out of my head and feel less hopeless.

Take It Further

Direction: Work in your learning community to reflect on, discuss, and answer the questions below.

1. Revisit the eight cases where neutrality is considered earlier in this chapter. Work with a partner or in your group to explore how you might coach in each situation. What factors influence your decision? Which situations would you approach with neutrality? Why?
2. Visit the NBHWC and ICF competencies and codes of ethics. (Follow the links that are online at *www.guilford.com/lanier-materials.*) Explain a few of the important factors that will help you decide when to remain neutral.
3. Read the comment from Coach Holly (below). Discuss this with a partner and explore other possible ways you might, or might not, use the decisional balance tool.

   > "To me, as a coach, I probably wouldn't use the decisional balance tool if I were coaching as part of a collaborative care team, where the goal is to get the patient to follow the prescription because, as the coach, I do have somewhat of an agenda. But as an independent coach, I find that this tool can be really effective at having some meaningful conversations about change."
   >
   > —COACH HOLLY, an NBHWC-certified Health and Wellness coach (personal communication, 2023)

4. What are some coaching situations that might call for you to choose to influence a client a particular way? How is MI-consistent coaching used in these situations?

Chapter 12

Planting Seeds of Discrepancy

It's a reasonable assumption that clients seek coaching because they desire and need to change or grow. Clients choose what to change—as in all coaching conversations—and you coach them toward their chosen agenda, not your agenda. In Chapter 11 we discussed situations where coaches choose neutrality when helping clients decide between two or more challenging options. Here, we explore ways to help those clients who do not have an expressed desire or need to change and are in the precontemplative stage of change. These clients are not ambivalent in at least one area, and you may hear little or no change talk to evoke. (See "The Stages of Change" in Chapter 5.)

This seeming contradiction raises the questions: "Then, why do they seek coaching?" and, more importantly, "What can I do to support them?" This chapter explores certain coaching conditions where you might cultivate some ambivalence for those who do not have any in one particular area.

Skilled coaches look for the "story under the story" and sometimes discover that clients who appear unmotivated are, in fact, ambivalent beneath the surface. What you perceive as the client's satisfaction with the status quo may be a defense against being scolded or lectured, or it could be self-protection from discomfort over failed attempts. Part of them wants a change, and the gap between intention and behavior may be too large or painful to consider. Coaching with MI is called for here, and you will use good listening, engaging, and evoking as you search for ambivalence. Tending to the environment first will prepare the soil for the seeds of ambivalence to germinate and grow.

WHEN CLIENTS HAVE NO AMBIVALENCE

But, even so, some clients will genuinely have no seeds of ambivalence to nourish, even buried under the surface. White and Miller (2007) reminded us that confrontation by arguing or persuading is ineffective in counseling, and we assert that it is equally ineffective in coaching. When people seem oblivious to what you and others see, and they persist in habits or thinking patterns that block growth, it can be tempting to shrug and hope that one day, after suffering enough, they become motivated. But they sit in front of you, and whether they are referred by a third party or come on their own, you have an opportunity. Motivation can be planted and nourished—within a trusting relationship—and this is your job as a coach.

Ambivalence requires an awareness of discrepancies between what is desired or valued and the current reality. Part of your work as a coach might be offering information that could raise questions about the status quo and illuminate a widening gap. As discussed in Chapter 8, there are ways to provide key pieces of information either that open the door for exploration or that shut down any consideration of change. Just-in-time information, given in the spirit of the coaches' CAPE and within your scope of practice and ethical boundaries, can help to open the door for exploration and initiate ambivalence.

Clients mandated by sponsors or stakeholders might be aware of and agree to the need for change but disagree with one or more of the specified areas of change. For example, a medical practitioner prescribes a diet, some exercise, and stress management techniques and emphasizes that the diet should be a priority. Yet once you begin working with the client, you discover that they do not see a need for change in their diet.

Below are some situations where clients seek coaching but do not have ambivalence; they lack reasons, desires, or a need to change in one area. As precontemplators, they are not aware or do not agree that a particular change is necessary.

- A school superintendent provides paid professional leave for coaching sessions, specifically for teachers who consistently have low-performing students.
- A parent hires a coach for their daughter, so she can get motivated to complete missing assignments and pass 11th grade.
- A business provides an employee incentive benefit for coaching because morale is low and workers are not performing as team players.
- An employee seeks coaching after a mark of "needs improvement" on a quarterly performance review but is unaware of which area to improve.
- Clients who report being "happy with their weight" are referred by

a physician to work on weight reduction, exercise, and stress management.

ACCEPTANCE WITHIN DISCREPANCY

How do you balance accepting where clients are and coaching toward their agenda while also raising awareness of the gap between the ideal and the current reality? How do you plant the seeds of ambivalence where none can be found? Part of your work is to help clients envision their desired future, life purpose, and values that shape that purpose. This is the work of evoking.

Discrepancy is the gap between this larger desired future and the current behavior. If the status quo does not conflict with something your client values more, then MI has no traction to work. A client's intrinsic motivations—their highest vision, purpose, and values—must be viewed in comparison to the current situation. You can cultivate ambivalence within your clients only as they perceive the change as something that will align with their values.

As you help clients explore that gap, remember that change becomes possible when people accept themselves just as they are. Self-acceptance frees people to consider the possibility of a discrepancy without inciting defensiveness that could stall things before they even start. Furthermore, when you, as a coach, demonstrate acceptance, you contribute to your client's freedom to explore discrepancies. Acceptance does not imply that you approve or agree with them. An enlarged view of acceptance outlined in Chapter 3 includes the coaches' CAPE elements of accurate empathy, honoring autonomy, demonstrating absolute worth, and offering affirmations.

Along with acceptance, you will also affirm your client's strengths and positive qualities. But eliciting their own self-discovery and articulation of these strengths and qualities may be more powerful than your affirmations. Research on self-affirmation has shown that it can minimize a person's defensive response to threats (Critcher et al., 2010).

INSTILLING DISCREPANCY

Flower farmers have a trade secret for nudging seeds to germinate early; "cold stratification" is designed to break dormancy and mimic natural seasonal changes. The farmer artificially subjects the seeds to winter's cold, damp conditions so they soften and burst open. Instilling discrepancy is similar. You are not inserting something into the person but you are curating the environment, so the conditions favor an initiation of discrepancy, which primes the consideration of growth.

Cultivating discrepancy is possible as you sit with your client—CAPE fastened—to consider the reasons why they *might* consider a change. The P in CAPE is essential as you remember the coaching relationship is an equal partnership and that "instilling" is a respectful process of infusion, done in a nonconfrontational way.

Explore What the Person Already Knows

When someone seems to lack information, and you hear very little change talk, this may tempt you to use "fixer" tools. But arguing and pushing are not helpful in the precontemplation phase. Before offering new information, starting with what clients already know is wise. Instead of you providing knowledge, exploring what they already know allows clients to voice that knowledge themselves.

If you offer information, use the ask–offer–ask strategy from Chapter 8 as a way of planting seeds. Approach with a hypothetical posture, ask permission, give small chunks (not buckets) of information, follow up with the last "A" to check on understanding, keep it brief, and most importantly, wear your CAPE. This approach prompts you to offer compassion, acceptance (in all its forms), partnership, and empowerment. The empowerment comes with your clear delivery of questions that help shift dormancy and nudge the seeds of ambivalence to germinate.

Here is an example of planting the seeds of discrepancy in a client who does not believe she needs to change her methods of instruction:

TEACHER: My principal sent me for coaching because my students' achievement scores are low. I don't think there's a problem with my instruction methods; it's because she keeps giving me students who struggle academically. But you're going to tell me what I should do, right?

COACH: Having struggling students is a real challenge for a teacher, for sure. So, what do you already know about how to increase students' achievement scores? [*Ask.*]

TEACHER: Well, if they had better scores, I'd look like a more effective teacher. (*Laughs.*)

COACH: That's true. Anything else?

TEACHER: I know checking progress at midterm exams is a little late to find out my students aren't learning the material. But I don't have time to test all day, every day, and anyway, with my students, I don't see what else I could do to help them improve their scores. [*The teacher seems to have little or no ambivalence.*]

COACH: Yes, it's true that frequent checks can help you adjust your teaching methods in time to boost student performance. What do you know about other things, like increasing active engagement to improve scores? [*Open question and offer.*]

TEACHER: You mean getting students to be involved in daily lessons? Yeah, I know that's supposed to help them learn. [*The teacher already has some knowledge.*]

COACH: That's right. Making sure your students are fully engaged in each lesson raises the likelihood that they'll learn. How does that align with what you know? [*Offer and ask, and developing discrepancy.*]

TEACHER: In every lesson? Well, I have a very unmotivated group this year, but I guess that makes sense. If I could only figure out how to engage them more, that might make a difference. [*Change talk.*]

COACH: What else do you know? [*Ask.*]

TEACHER: Some teachers do small-group instruction, and that's supposed to help students learn. But then again, you need excellent classroom management for that to work, and with a class like mine, with 28 academically diverse students, that's hard to do. I guess if I could do that, I might be able to increase their active engagement and get them more motivated to learn. [*Client has some knowledge. Coach planted seeds for change talk.*]

COACH: You have a challenging class, and it sounds like you may want small-group instruction to raise their engagement. If you want, I can tell you how to arrange small groups and then show you some strategies for building active engagement. [*Ask, offer, reflect change talk.*]

TEACHER: Sure, I'd like that. I really do want to help my students learn. [*Change talk.*]

COACH: That's why you're in the business, right? I want that, too.

Explore Others' Concerns

Clients sometimes lack concern about a particular issue but are referred for coaching because of others' concerns. You can help expand their awareness to see "what is" and, in this way, plant seeds for change as they rethink and reconsider new perspectives. It's the client's privilege and responsibility to do something with the discoveries, and it's your role to refrain from the "fixing reflex" while you allow space for the client to make sense of what others know. Remain curious, listen deeply, and avoid stacked questions that sound like a clinical-style inquisition. Within this awareness, clients see another's perspective or consider new information that can initiate consideration of change. As a result, you may hear change talk emerge.

As we said, the partnership component of the coaches' CAPE is an essential consideration, since sharing others' concerns—when your client does not share the same concern—can be an uncomfortable conversation.

Remain flexible and present with your client as you invite their active voice to direct the session. When choices are offered, remember the decision belongs to the client. Your main job within this partnership, even while providing others' concerns, is to be curious, observant, focused, and nonjudgmental. MI-consistent coaching invites clients to reflect on their lives in a container of acceptance and safety as they consider a change.

Following is a coaching example of a client who does not share the perspective of a concerned "other." Notice how the coach plants seeds for change.

COACH: What do you think your mother worries about with your schoolwork? [*Open question.*]

CLIENT: She's always on my case about it, and I think she needs to let me make my own decisions, especially since I'm in the 11th grade. Her lectures and nagging just make me feel worse. I don't see the big deal; at least, I don't think it's worth all the fighting.

COACH: Your mother seems to be overreacting about this, and it annoys you. You're capable of making your own decisions. [*Amplified reflection, reflects sustain talk.*]

CLIENT: Well, maybe not overreacting. I guess she wants to make sure I graduate high school. But she's annoying me for sure. I mean, there are other things way more important than this, and she doesn't seem to understand and appreciate me. She kept nagging me about schoolwork I missed when I was out for a month in the fall, and I never made it up, and now I've got an academic warning or something. I'm ready to move on, and she's treating me like a kid.

COACH: Why do you suppose she's nagging you? [*Open question with curiosity.*]

CLIENT: Well, I guess she wants me to pass 11th grade. She's worried I'll just quit school if I have to go to summer school. (*Laughs.*) She's probably right about that; I've never liked school and just want to be done. But no one else in my family quit school, and that worries her that I wouldn't finish. She's always talking about what kind of job I might get in the future.

COACH: A few of the things bothering her are that you might have to go to summer school, which may cause you to drop out of school and not graduate, and that, in turn, would limit your future opportunities for getting a good job. What else might she be thinking about? [*Summary and offering a small chunk of information.*]

CLIENT: Maybe she doesn't want me to depend on someone else. She's a single mother, and when I was a kid, she always told me I needed to learn to stand on my own two feet. I guess I can see her point in a way; I mean, everyone says you need a good education to get a good job.

Note: The coach reflects some sustain talk in the above example. Sometimes, when you do this, it elicits the opposite perspective, especially in the context of the concerns of a loved one.

Offering Your Own or Others' Expertise

Another way to develop discrepancy when people seem to lack ambivalence is to gather more information from your expertise or a reliable source. Clients in the precontemplative stage may have misunderstandings that prevent them from recognizing a potential growth point. For example, suppose a client believes counting calories is most important and claims that calories from a croissant equal the calories from a plate of leafy greens and colorful vegetables. In that case, you may need to provide more information about the vast differences in the nutritional value of each.

The NBHWC scope of practice guidelines (2021) state that coaches can provide expert guidance if they hold nationally recognized credentials. You can also offer resources from nationally recognized authorities such as the Centers for Disease Control and Prevention and the American College of Lifestyle Medicine. Regardless of the source, your empathic delivery of information or suggestions can stimulate consideration of change. Here's an example.

CLIENT: The doctor is concerned about my body mass index and something about my waist measurement being too big.

COACH: What do you think about his concern? [*Open question.*]

CLIENT: He says it's about my risk of heart disease. But like I told him, I just have one of those pear-shaped bodies. It doesn't matter if I lose weight; I will still have this belly. It has nothing to do with heart disease.

COACH: I have some information on that topic that I could share if you like. [*Ask.*]

CLIENT: Sure, if you think there's something I'm missing.

COACH: Are you familiar with the Centers for Disease Control and Prevention?

CLIENT: Yeah, I know about the CDC. Do they have something to say about my waist size?

COACH: A large waistline, along with high blood pressure, which you have, and a high triglyceride level are three factors that put you at risk for metabolic syndrome. [*Offer.*]

CLIENT: And what is metabolic syndrome?

COACH: Metabolic syndrome is the name for a group of factors that raises your risk for heart disease and other health problems, like diabetes and stroke. Is there anything else you'd like to know? [*Offer, ask.*]

CLIENT: You mean my waist size is a problem? [*Consideration of a reason to change.*]

Collecting Feedback

Often, your clients who do not seem ambivalent can gain access to information that awakens a consideration to find out more. Clients are more likely to explore possibilities when you encourage an experimental mindset and avoid insisting on a commitment. When clients have access to assessment feedback such as lab testing or norm-referenced biomarker data, it can promote discrepancy and motivation to at least consider a change. Assessments can give a snapshot and provide comparisons that may be helpful to encourage discrepancy and the motivation to consider change (Brown, 1998; Reid et al., 2010). The result can be change talk in people who were unsure they had a problem.

If you have invested time in engaging and cultivating trust in a nonjudgmental relationship, you can provide feedback or use the MI method of ask–offer–ask to provide information and feedback if your clients are open to it. Here is an example of a session after the client agreed to track her heart rate with a wearable tracking device.

COACH: Last week, you mentioned that you didn't think stress impacted you very much. In fact, you didn't think it was that big of a concern. What did you learn from tracking your heart rate this week?

CLIENT: Oh wow! I had no idea how much my heart rate changed, and it looks like it might be related to stress. I did like you said, and I checked it six times a day and wrote the numbers down on a graph. When I was in meetings, my heart rate would increase, which I expected. But what surprised me was it stayed elevated for a long time afterward. [*Awareness of discrepancy.*]

COACH: That's quite a discovery. What else did you notice?

CLIENT: Well, I also started meditation this week, right after my lunch breaks. And every single time, my heart rate went down lower than it's been in a very long time. My doctor warned me that I had to control my stress, and I think I understand what he meant. What do you think this has to do with my high blood pressure? [*The question implies permission to offer information.*]

COACH: When you're relaxed, as in your meditation practice, your heart rate and blood pressure lower. And the opposite is true; in times of stress, your body will respond with raised blood pressure, heart rate, and breathing. Your doctor has asked you to manage your stress responses as much as possible. What do you think about that information? [*Offer and ask.*]

CLIENT: So, you're saying stress really does have something to do with my high blood pressure?

Another good start when change talk is not coming is to ask, "Take me through a typical day." Directional questions can uncover behavior patterns or shifts in energy, and a discussion of areas of concern may emerge naturally. Your intended outcome is ambivalence, which will indicate that your client is moving toward the consideration of change.

Reframing

Reframing, previously addressed in Chapter 4, may be another way to plant seeds for change by offering a different meaning or exploring another perspective about what the person currently knows or assumes. Reframing is done casually, without direct attention and emphasis, and you use reflections followed by open questions to raise awareness and new perspectives. Here's an example of a client whose doctor has ordered her to manage stress, but she currently blames her coworker for the stress.

CLIENT: Like I said, my doctor suggested I start meditation before taking medicine, but I don't think I have a problem with stress. I have high blood pressure because it's hereditary, and there's not much I can do about it. The real problem is a coworker I'm supposed to help, but she's making it difficult with all her interruptions. [*No ambivalence.*]

COACH: Being interrupted in your day makes things difficult for you. [*Reflection, not an attempt to correct her.*]

CLIENT: Yes, she didn't know what to do this week, and my supervisor told me to help her. She's the most disorganized person in the world, and I can't understand why she doesn't do what I say and get her work done, and that's what's causing my stress. [*Long story about the coworker.*] She needs me, but I have more responsibilities at work now, and I'm already overloaded.

COACH: You're too busy to help her. As you talk, I notice an energy shift. What are you experiencing right now? [*Reflection of emotion.*]

CLIENT: (*Pauses.*) Well, my heart's racing, I'm a little tense, I feel tight right here (*Points to shoulders*), and I'm sweating. My heart is pounding so much I feel it in my chest and can hear pounding in my ears. I really don't like this.

COACH: This sounds like what you and your doctor discussed. What about your response would you like to change? [*Not insisting on a new perspective but planting a seed and offering.*]

CLIENT: About me? What do I want to change about myself? (*Coach nods.*) Well, I guess we *are* talking about me, aren't we? (*Laughs.*) Yeah, I get it; this is *my* stress response, isn't it?

COACH: What you're experiencing sounds like a stress response, yes. What's your understanding of stress now? [*Coach refrains from adding more information. Exploring what client already knows, planting seeds.*]

CLIENT: I think it's less about my coworker and maybe more about how I respond to her. We've talked about how I have choices, and I think this may be one of those times. [*Client reframes and considers a new perspective.*]

In some instances, you may find no ambivalence, and there seems to be nothing to evoke. The ground appears stiff, and the seeds are dormant. If you poke too much and in the wrong way, you may get pushback and risk causing the person to remain in the status quo. We find that taking time to prepare the soil first and then gently planting a few seeds allows the client to consider a change. This may not happen immediately but might happen further down the road. Honor your client's power to make their own decisions, avoid confrontation, and allow the process to unfold, holding the door open for a future return to the issue.

Coaching Sample: Planting Seeds

This is an example of coaching when the client had little to no ambivalence around the prescribed plan. Notice how the coach softens discord to reengage the client.

The coach, the client, and the referring physician made prior agreements for a team approach. The coach's role was to help the client implement the mandated protocols and provide information and education if needed while spending most of the time in the coach approach.

COACH: Your doctor sent over this plan, and there are several things here, and he asks you first to change your diet for 3 weeks. What part of your diet would you like to work on in our session today? [*Coach assumes a target for the session.*]

CLIENT: Well, hold on a minute. I knew I had to make changes, but I didn't agree to change my diet. What kinds of things do I have to eliminate? [*Hints of discord.*]

COACH: It says here sugar, sweets, gluten, and dairy, along with alcohol and caffeine. I think you and your doctor were looking for some causes for your symptoms.

CLIENT: Well, if you take away the sweets and goodies I bake for my family, you're taking away my happiness. I don't want to do that, and I don't know if I could. [*Discord.*]

COACH: I notice a strong reaction to this. What is this bringing up for you?

CLIENT: I feel like I need to change and get healthier, sure; that's why I went to see the doctor and signed up for coaching. But I probably didn't read the list of things very carefully, and gosh, this is too overwhelming for me right now.

COACH: I'm sorry if I pushed you. You're feeling it's asking too much. [*Apology, reestablishing the partnership, reflecting meaning.*]

CLIENT: Yes, it is! Things have been hard for me lately, and if you throw me too many things all at once, I will probably fail and then quit. My job is way too stressful to stop things and try to change this *big* thing.

COACH: I understand. As your coach, I'm here to help you achieve what you want. What do you feel would be in your best interest here? You're in charge of what you do. [*Coaches' CAPE. The client has no apparent ambivalence about the diet but may be open to considering other areas.*]

CLIENT: I know I'm being difficult. Can I be honest?

COACH: Please do.

CLIENT: If I don't get my house clutter cleaned out, I can't get my kids or me to where we have to go on time. We're always looking for lost things and having all this stuff in my daily life is an intrusion. (*Takes a deep breath, pauses.*)

COACH: It's zapping all your energy to have the clutter. [*Amplified reflection.*] So, for today, it sounds like you want to work on decluttering your house first. Is that right?

CLIENT: Definitely! I'm tapped out, and I might feel better if I could just organize my house, closets, and drawers. Who knows, once I do that, it might be possible for me to do that special diet for 3 weeks. [*The softer approach helped the client consider changing her diet. The coach avoids reactance by not confronting.*]

Yeah, that makes me feel better, just tackling this one thing, and then we'll see what happens after that. Do you think we need to ask my doctor first?

COACH: Sure, let him know your choice about what you want to do first. So, for today what would you like to accomplish by the end of our meeting? [*Clarify and refocus.*]

CLIENT: I want to list everything I need to get cleaned out and make a timeline for getting that done.

COACH: You've got a starting point. What else may have come to mind that would be helpful to explore so you can get all you need today? [*Soft invitation and planting of seeds of ambivalence.*]

CLIENT: Well, maybe you could explain more about this diet. I mean, I'm open to at least reading about it. It'll be hard for me because a lot is happening, and my husband and kids are not on board with changing anything about our eating. And I don't have time like I said.

I didn't mean to be so dramatic earlier; it just caught me off guard, that's all. I don't know if you noticed, but I was about to hyperventilate! (*Long pause.*) I do want to feel better and have more energy, and this diet issue has been in the back of my mind for a while. I know it's the hardest thing to tackle, and I want to have some success in something else first, and then I might be brave enough to work on the diet. [*A mix of sustain and change talk, ambivalence.*]

Notice that the coach planted the seeds of ambivalence slowly and gently after responding to the discord. This example demonstrates that a lack of ambivalence in one area does not mean clients are unwilling to change in another. A good lesson from this coaching sample is to not make assumptions. The client was not ambivalent—yet—about the diet but was in the planning stage of change in decluttering her house. The hope is that within an MI-consistent coaching container, you can plant seeds of ambivalence so clients begin to imagine, explore, and plan a way forward.

The Rest of the Story

The seeds of ambivalence planted early in the coaching relationship of the sample dialogue above later germinated and produced a change in many areas of this client's life. After cleaning her closets, she felt empowered to tackle the 3-week elimination diet. At the end of the 3-week diet, many symptoms resolved, and she felt motivated to keep some dietary changes as part of her daily routine. A few months later, she reduced many medications and entirely reversed most of her symptoms. At the end of 3 months, she achieved all her goals, including improved relationships and less stress in her job. Her improvements and changes have been long-lasting. A year later, she reported flourishing as an energetic, healthy, and emotionally available woman for her family, friends, and employers. (As a bonus, her family also adopted her healthy way of eating!)

Take It Further

Directions: Work in your learning community or with a partner to read and discuss your answers to the questions below.

1. How can the CAPE (demonstrating acceptance for your clients) help build a client's exploration and discovery of a discrepancy between their ideal and the current reality?
2. What might be some benefits of affirming client strengths and positive traits when ambivalence is lacking?
3. This chapter explores five ways you, as a coach, could plant seeds of discrepancy for those clients who seem to have no ambivalence. Define and explain those five ways.

Chapter 13

The Planning Task

Effective coaching with MI includes developing clear goals and detailed plans for reaching them (Miller & Moyers, 2021). In focusing, we discussed the "what" of change (Chapter 5), then in evoking, we examined the "why" of change (Chapter 6), and here in planning, we address the "how" of change. How do you know when to shift from talking about the "why" of change to the "how" of change? What role do you, as coach, play, and how can you use your expertise when your clients need it?

Keep your coaches' CAPE tied all through planning to remind yourself of the way to do what you do. Continue your engaging skills as you focus on clients' chosen change goals. This helps you avoid becoming overly focused on the "how" and losing sight of the "who" in front of you. Remember, you coach the person, not the problem.

Planning is a continuation of evoking, and those same MI skills are used here to elicit ideas for how to change. As you did in focusing, you move from general to specific, from long- or short-term goals to smaller action steps. For example, being motivated to "get healthy" is a broad concept that needs specific steps. A good place to start is to circle back and recall a client's larger vision before moving on to the specifics of what they want to do. The small, achievable action steps are tied to that broader view.

TRANSITION FROM EVOKING TO PLANNING

Evoking the why of change generally comes before planning the how, although the tasks overlap. Be cautious; after engaging and focusing, avoid skipping evoking and rushing straight to planning. Doing so can tend toward goal management instead of coaching. Although some clients may be ready to take this direct route, most will benefit from the evoking task, and you continue those skills as you transition to planning. Clients who developed a plan before they were ready may report a less-than-successful experience on their follow-up visit. Planning for action is, in some ways, a natural progression from talking about why to change to talking about how to go about changing.

Some Signs of Readiness

After listening well (engaging) and discussing the "what" (focusing) and "why" (evoking), there comes a time to consider the "how" of change. How do you know if there is enough "why" to talk about how change might happen? Often, it occurs naturally, and you hear indications of readiness as the client talks or asks about how change could happen.

Recall the MI hill of change in Chapter 6. Navigating through engaging, focusing, and evoking can seem like an uphill climb in facilitating a person's reasons for change, but planning can be a smoother, downhill journey. Occasionally, some clients explicitly affirm readiness by saying, "I'm ready to go! Let's get started!" However, many are still somewhat reluctant and ambivalent about change. You can hone your listening skills to hear movement toward change, whether it's a firm commitment—"I will stop drinking alcohol tonight, and that is final!"—or a more subtle leaning toward, "I'd love to have a life without headaches." As you evoke on the far side of the hill, the mobilizing side, notice change talk that indicates movement toward planning.

The most obvious sign is that you hear more change talk and less sustain talk. Other than that, as you listen and focus on the *who* of the session, not just the *what,* you may notice a shift in energy where the client seems to embrace a more peaceful and calm state, indicating acceptance of the imagined future. You may sense quietness as they focus energy on designing a path for moving forward.

As the envisioned future becomes clearer for clients, they may ask about change and even generate some ideas on how they would take steps to achieve what they want. Your client is envisioning a desired state and, in this way, role-playing positive outcomes. They may state this vision positively or negatively, as both are about a possible change. As we said, reluctance and ambivalence may remain, and envisioning can almost seem like a type of reluctance, imagining the change and potential challenges. You may hear this expressed in questions about how, when, and what if.

> "How would I fit this new work assignment into my schedule?"
>
> "If I stopped scolding my teenager, she might listen to me about other things."

BOX 13.1. Signs of Readiness to Change

1. An increase in ***change talk,*** the desire, ability, reasons, and needs to change.
2. A decrease in ***sustain talk.***
3. A peaceful and calm state, a feeling of ***resolve.***
4. ***Envisioning or imagining*** what change (or the challenges of change) might be like.
5. ***Direct questions*** about the specifics of how change can happen.
6. Talk about taking small and achievable steps that lead to client success.

"What if I threw away my sweets but then had a sugar craving?"
"How could I possibly do this with what I have going on?"
"What if my family doesn't like what I cook?"
"When would I fit in exercise since I work 60 hours a week?"

These questions may reveal lingering doubts or obstacles, or clients may simply need assistance unpacking all the details of a plan. MI-consistent coaching helps you guide your clients toward resolving these questions to achieve success. (See Box 13.1 for a list of some signs of readiness to change.)

As people consider a new change, it's normal to hear them envisioning what this might be like and talking out the pros and cons. Listen for mobilizing change talk as the internal committee considers the "how" of change. You may hear signs of moving from the preparation to the contemplation stage of change.

You may hear some sustain talk as they anticipate challenges, such as "But it feels impossible sometimes," or "But if I took a stand, would she still want to be friends with me?" Preparing for change can happen incrementally over time, and your evoking skills are needed here to shine a light on the next step in the journey.

TESTING THE WATER

There are ways to find out if your client is ready to discuss the how of change. Strong signals sound like "I'm absolutely going to do this," "I'm going to do whatever it takes," or "Yes, I'm ready to get started!" But softer signals are equally important and can indicate some level of commitment and activation to plan, "I could probably do that," "It's pretty likely," and "I'll give it some thought."

As you hear mobilizing change talk emerge, even slightly, be encouraged and patiently inquire. Consider how your expertise is needed as you partner with your client for success. Respond with curiosity about what strengths, skills, and characteristics they could use to help them move forward. Even the slightest efforts to move toward change warrant celebration, affirmation, and optimism.

CLIENT: I probably need to keep track of what I eat. If not, I forget, and my eating gets out of control. [*Reasons to change. Activation language.*]

COACH: What are you considering for a way to keep track of your eating?

CLIENT: I thought a food journal could show me how much unhealthy food I eat. I could at least see how much is in my diet. [*Tentative change talk.*]

COACH: What benefits do you think you'd gain from this journal? [*Evoking more change talk.*]

CLIENT: If I was brave enough to write it down, it might make me more able to commit to doing better. Writing things down seems to make things more official. [*Change talk.*]

COACH: You've mentioned before that bravery is one of your highest strengths. What other characteristics do you have that you want to call upon to help you with the food journal?

CLIENT: Well, if I did the journal, it might be one more thing on my to-do list, even though it would keep me accountable. Maybe I should think of something more feasible for me. [*Considering pros and cons.*]

COACH: This is important to you, and you want to find something that works. You definitely know what works best for you. [*Partnering.*]

Summarizing

One standard MI way to test the water is to summarize all the change talk you heard and offer it back as a bouquet.

> "You envision more energy and fulfillment if you had a balanced approach to work. You'd feel like spending time with your kids and be motivated to return to fun things like hiking and playing tennis with your friends. You want to enjoy life again and return to the 'real you,' the one you've put on hold during this 2-year project. I notice an excitement in your voice when you talk about all the possibilities."

Summarizing is one of the core MI skills, and in planning, summaries should be used to forward momentum. Recall that in the evoking task, OARS skills are strategically used to ask about, affirm, reflect, and summarize all the change talk. Since planning is an extension of the evoking task, you will use this type of directional summary here.

While various types of summaries serve different purposes, the most important one for planning is one that asks for more change talk. We see three types of summaries in MI-consistent coaching conversations (see Figure 13.1).

1. A summary could focus on feelings, especially negative emotions. This type of summary might help to build empathy and rapport, especially early in the session, but this kind of summary lacks the goal-oriented component of evoking. If helpers use this type of summary in the planning task, clients are not likely to go anywhere.

2. Some summaries capture both sides of someone's ambivalence, both sustain talk and change talk. Simply reflecting and offering back all your client says might demonstrate good listening and recall, but it lacks the directional movement needed in the planning task. Furthermore, this kind of summary will likely reinforce ambivalence, not resolve it. In planning, continue to wear your coaches' CAPE to empower your clients' commitment to and creative plans for change.

3. As we said earlier, the ideal MI summary in the planning task pulls in most of the change talk and offers it back to the client as a bouquet. It is strategic and consciously directed toward change—for example:

> "So, here's what you've said so far. You want more balance in your drinking and eating habits on the weekend. You're hoping this will prevent the Monday morning 'slump' and low energy you feel and also probably alleviate the 'guilt' you have after overindulging on the weekends. You want to go from a 60/40 ratio of good habits to more like an 80/20 balance of healthy eating and drinking overall."

1. Summary of feelings, and negative emotions.	⤸	You may connect with your client, but this lacks the goal-oriented component of evoking.
2. Summary captures both sides of change talk in summary.	⟺	This may show you're listening well, but it lacks the directional movement needed in evoking task.
3. Summary pulls in most of the change talk offered.	⟹	This is the quintessential MI summary. It is strategic, and consciously directed toward change.

FIGURE 13.1. Three types of summaries.

You will want to refrain from offering commentary when giving a summary, since it could interrupt the focus and flow of a client's ideas. As you do throughout the session, keep your recapitulation brief and concise. Be careful to limit the sustain talk statements in your summary so you do not encourage the con side of the argument. Some coaches choose not to include any sustain talk in this recap summary.

The Key Question

After a summary to recap the person's own desire, ability, reason, and need to change, you ask a short and simple question about what is needed next. This key question evokes forward movement toward change. A key question for the example above might be: "So, after considering all of that, what do you think you'll do?" Here are other examples of key questions.

- "So far, what sounds like a feasible plan?"
- "What's the next step you might be considering?"
- "How do you think you'll proceed?"

These key questions highlight how you can effectively guide and structure a session while respecting your clients' freedom to choose the direction and approach of the plan.

Another way to check on readiness is to ask directly in the form of a scaling question. As described in Chapter 7, you could ask how "important" a change is on a scale of 1 to 10 or how "confident" your client is to do it. We do not recommend asking how "ready" your client is, since this can feel too pushy, as if you were asking for a commitment. You want your clients to reach their own conclusions after reflecting on importance and confidence.

Avoid Pressuring

Asking for a commitment (e.g., "What are you going to do?") could pressure the client prematurely and spark defensiveness. Instead, you might offer something less demanding, such as "What do you think you might like to do?" Open the door for your client, but step aside as they choose to walk through on their own.

Offer the Gift of Space and Time

In a typical chat among friends, two or more voices overlap, with one beginning before the other has finished. This mingled stream of voices is part of the rhythm of conversation, but coaching is not chatting. In coaching, your goal is to create the space where clients can delve deeper into their thoughts and emotions, reflect, reconsider their thinking, and vocalize their ideas. Ultimately, clients should envision a way forward toward change (Kimsey-House et al., 2018).

Creating this space requires a coach to be silent and comfortable with long pauses, which demands strong self-management. This MI-consistent approach is especially warranted when you are tempted to fix your client or think you know what they need (NBHWC, 2022). If you feel hurried and find you are working hard, check in with yourself to see how fully you trust the coaching process. Furthermore, observe how well you embody the MI belief that your client is creative and resourceful and can solve their own problems. After the key question, practice patience as your client takes time to consider what to do.

Resist the Fixing Reflex

Evoking the "why" of change on the preparatory side of the change hill can feel like hiking lateral trails with hairpin turns. The descent down the mobilizing side of the hill—the "how"—resembles coasting, but it's a time for caution. In your enthusiasm, resist becoming too directive and getting ahead of your client, since you know that a fixing reflex can squelch the motivation you cultivated earlier (Miller & Rollnick, 2023).

As we said, engaging is initiated early in the coaching relationship, and it describes the way of *being* with your client throughout this last task of planning. Engaging undergirds the entire coaching conversation as you continue to support your clients to uncover what works for them, even among remaining ambivalence.

Coaching Sample: Transitioning to Planning

CLIENT: I'm so tired of feeling bad, it feels overwhelming to think about changing how I eat, but I need to do something. It's discouraging to think of the times when I've tried and failed, but I'm 46 years old. My doctor scared me about what diabetes could mean to my future, so there was no time to make any more excuses. I want to be healthy and enjoy my teens while they're still home, but it feels impossible sometimes.	[*Increasing change talk, among ambivalence.*]
COACH: I sense some excitement in your voice about feeling better and possibly changing your eating patterns and, of	[*Reflect change talk.*]

course, enjoying your teens while they're still home.

CLIENT: You heard me right. I want this and know I'll feel a lot better, but sometimes, it's too much. [*Change talk, tentative change talk.*]

COACH: You still have concerns. What would it mean to not be afraid of making these changes? [*Reflect, followed by evoking question.*]

CLIENT: Hmm, good question. I guess it means I wouldn't get stuck; I could go forward. But I'm responsible for cooking for my family, and if I did change my eating, how would I do it with all that? Don't get me wrong. I'm here because I fully intend to change and know I need it. As I said, the blood work scares me, and I'm afraid of what could happen. But, to answer your question, I guess it would feel more doable if I could ease into it slowly; maybe that would help. What do you think? [*Change talk, questions about how. Subtle signs of readiness to plan.*]

COACH: You're considering how to make it work, and one thing you're thinking about is easing into the change slowly. What are some examples of easing into this slowly? [*Reflecting, followed by directional evoking (asking for examples).*]

CLIENT: I don't like to do anything halfway, so I need more planning time to do this right. Maybe another week to think and journal about this and plan for how to talk to my kids. My husband is usually supportive, but my kids won't understand. [*Devising an action plan, one that is feasible and personalized.*]

COACH: You put a lot of thought into a plan. What do you imagine this plan will look like? [*Affirmation, evoking details of the plan.*]

CLIENT: Ah! I know what to do! We have a weekend getaway coming up, and I think this would be the perfect spot to have a conversation with everyone. I can journal about it first and make sure I know what I want to say. Yeah, that's a good plan. [*Envisioning, imagining, taking steps, and developing specifics of the plan. Shift in energy.*]

COACH: You sound sure and excited! What will it look like if your family talk goes just like you want?	[*Affirming, evoking, envisioning.*]
CLIENT: Well, ideally, they'll all hug me and say, "We support you!" (*Laughs.*) But realistically, we need to talk about options. (*Pause*) My teens can cook, so maybe there's a way for them to be involved.	[*Envisioning a feasible plan. A calm, quiet mood.*]
COACH: What would be important for you as you have this conversation?	[*Connect larger values to action steps.*]
CLIENT: If I had my family on board, I'd feel more comfortable making a menu and shopping for a new way of eating. I'm not as anxious when I hear myself saying that, and it feels good to think I'm close to making such a significant change.	[*Client talked herself into change. The possibilities are forming. Shift in energy, resolve.*]
COACH: You've wanted this change for a long time. What will you do after we get off the call to get ready to talk to your family?	[*Evoking forwarding momentum.*]
CLIENT: Well, I could plan for it. Do you think that'll work, or should I do this without having this talk? I'm afraid they might discourage me.	[*Tentative commitment language.*]
COACH: What feels like it will help you the most?	[*Honor autonomy.*]
CLIENT: I'm going to think on it first, and then journal some thoughts about it in the morning. I already have a journal. When we're all together this weekend, I'll be ready for a family chat.	[*Stronger commitment language; taking steps.*]
COACH: You're making some major changes, and you plan to think, journal, and then have a family talk. I sense your optimism for starting. What else do you think you'll need?	[*Brief summary of change talk, and an evoking key question.*]
CLIENT: Yes, I'm pretty excited about it. I don't think I need anything else right now. I can do the journaling and meditating right away.	[*Commitment language, clear plan.*]

SHARING INFORMATION AND ADVICE

To say that clients are experts in their own lives does not imply that you withhold information or advice that they need and expect in the planning task. You may have relevant experiences and wisdom to share, along with a developed skill of intuition that is valuable to your clients. When you use an MI-consistent approach, you can offer your expertise in a way that keeps you in the scope of practice. You will have already outlined with your clients the distinctions between teaching, mentoring, therapy, consulting, and other forms of helping. After you explain what you do *not* do, you define what coaching *is,* what it can do for them, and what *you,* as a coach, can bring to the relationship.

A common client question in the planning task is "How do people do this?" or "How would I do this?" As mentioned earlier, clients often need more support during planning, which may come in the form of information, advice, intuition, or brainstorming ways to move forward. The most important thing to remember is *how* to share these things. You do not withhold what is in the client's best interest but you selectively offer information and advice in a way that minimizes pushback and reluctance.

This topic was covered more fully in Chapter 8, but here is a brief review of skillful ways to offer information and advice. In addition to these guidelines, remember that health and wellness coaches are advised by the NBHWC to offer information from evidence-based resources or nationally recognized authorities. Whether the information is from you or another resource, share it in an MI-consistent way.

Ask Permission

Take a respectful approach and first knock on the door, ensuring you have permission before offering anything. You may hear a direct request for advice or information, such as:

- "Is there anything else I should do?"
- "After I finish this plan, what should I do next?"

If you have not had a request from your client, you can ask direct permission to share before moving ahead with your offering. We use "offering" intentionally, since you present this to your client without condition or expectation (ICF core competency 7). They can take it or leave it, and in this way, you guard their fundamental need for self-determination and autonomy.

- "What do you need to know about time management?"
- "Would you be interested in hearing about a resource I have?"

Coaches also embody an MI-consistent mindset by becoming aware of and using their intuition to benefit clients. You can evoke awareness and learning by sharing your insights, intuitions, and observations in service of the client's awareness (ICF core competencies 1 and 7). Even here, it may be appropriate to ask permission before sharing.

- "I'm noticing a shift in your energy when you talk about this. May I share what I notice?"
- "May I share a bit about behavior change research that might impact your decision?"

Promote Autonomy

Maintain respect for clients' autonomy and decision-making abilities in the planning task. Sometimes this is communicated with a disclaimer: "The final decision is up to you, but I have some ideas for what other people found helpful. Would you like to hear some things that might work in your situation?" When you respect your clients' autonomy and phrase things as optional, you can combine this with asking permission.

Ask–Offer–Ask

Coaching is facilitating a learning journey for clients, and in planning, they often seek information and ask for your input. Collecting information is just the starting point of learning, but it's not enough on its own. Learning requires assimilating information in a way that is meaningful and relevant to the learner. Effective teachers do not assume that what they offer will be accepted, understood, and applied in novel situations. Hence, teachers provide information in small chunks and frequently pause to check for understanding. So, too, as an MI-consistent coach, you will use the ask–offer–ask (A-O-A) method to check in before and after offering a chunk of information or advice. You ask permission, provide a small chunk of information or advice, then follow up with another question to see if they understood and if they have further questions or reactions to what they heard. This cycle repeats in a way that becomes spontaneous and natural for the client. (See Chapter 8 for more information about this technique.)

Focus on the "Who"

As a coach, you listen for possibilities and a way forward, not for pathologies or problems to solve. An MI-consistent coaching approach believes people have their own motivations, are creative and resourceful, and can solve their problems. This sets the tone for the way you share information and advice. Merely listening for solutions can become a block to coaching because it imposes an agenda to find answers, often too soon (Williams & Menendez, 2015).

This approach clarifies the key element: Coaches coach individuals rather than addressing problems. Coaches coach the "who" rather than just the "what." When devising a plan and providing information, consider not just the specifics but also the persons involved. Reflect on how the plan (or information) will affect who they are and who they want to *be*. What will they gain from it? How significant is it to them and what is their level of confidence to achieve it? How closely does it align with their personal values and aspirations? When negotiating a specific goal with someone, first consider their overall well-being. Consider the person in their entirety.

Offer Choices

Learning and insight translate to action, which is the aim of planning. Coaching conversations during the evoking task explore the *why* of change, where clients become more aware of the gap between what is and what is desired. In planning, increasing clients' awareness of possibilities is critical, since awareness promotes choice. As the choices become more evident, clients feel more freedom to respond creatively to life's dilemmas rather than react to them. Choosing from various options is less threatening than a prescribed one-size-fits-all plan. For this reason, MI-consistent coaching offers a menu of options as you invite clients to consider the how of change. (See Chapter 8 for further details on providing choices.)

> "Yes, you could do quite a few things to manage your stress. Experts advise several effective things, but as I mention them, you can decide if there's anything in this list that you'd like to try for yourself. You could do a relaxation exercise like deep belly breathing twice a day, take a brisk walk, find ways to laugh, play soothing music, or use positive self-talk. Of those things, which ones, if any, would you like to consider?"

In Chapter 8, we suggested that presenting options without breaks in between is better than presenting them one at a time, because hearing options as a group eliminates any implicit pressure on clients to justify their decisions. When people freely choose what they want to do, they are more likely to be committed to it and follow through.

DESIGNING A CHANGE PLAN

In this final task of the coaching conversation, you partner with clients in creating plans, steps, and commitments to move forward and transform learning and insight into action. Setting a clear focus in the beginning leads to a productive ending. In this task, clients develop new skills and approaches that result in a variety of actions, which in turn promote growth.

General Guidelines

While there are numerous ways to negotiate plans, whether for learning or behavior goals, there are general guidelines to keep in mind as you coach in an MI-consistent way (Acha, 2023). Below is a list of four guidelines for a coach to consider in this planning task.

1. *Focus on presence.* Maintaining an MI-consistent *way* of being with clients is vital to the planning journey, and you keep your coaches' CAPE fastened all the way through the session. Here is a review of the components of the spirit of MI, which we call the coaches' CAPE.

   - *Compassion* demonstrates an intentional effort to understand and promote a client's ideas for moving forward, and you defer to what is in a client's best interest.
   - *Acceptance* involves your nonjudgmental respect for your clients' value as human beings and their ideas for reaching their desired future.
   - *Partnership* recognizes there are two experts in the relationship. You can offer your coaching expertise to help increase the chances of success, and you know that clients are experts in their own lives.
   - *Empowerment* emphasizes the importance of people's own strengths, motivations, and resourcefulness, especially as they choose how to achieve what they want. You promote client autonomy when you embody this spirit in the planning task.

2. *Provide structure.* It's your job as the coach to frame the conversation in a way that leads to forward momentum. Provide a transition as you move—in the middle of a session—from the evoking task to the planning task. Here are some examples.

   - "As you've been exploring ____________ [topic] today, what might be some possible ways you could move forward with the discoveries you've made?"
   - "What could you do to move forward with your plan/ideas?"

The skills of evoking continue in planning, and you use the OARS skills in a directional way to evoke more commitment language. Move from broad to specific in the conversation. A discussion about change plans often begins with longer-range goals, then focuses on mid-range goals, and then moves to specific steps in the immediate future that will lead to attaining those more distant goals. The terminology varies among coaches, and we encourage you to use language that your clients understand. For example, a long-range goal, such as "lose 30 pounds in 6 months," cannot be accomplished in a day, but require several steps to achieve it. Some call these "action steps" or short-term goals. Regardless of the terminology used, help your clients put their plans into the context of the broader picture. A goal is most motivating if it is tied to a larger vision, which includes meaning, purpose, and even dreams of an ideal future.

3. *Use an experimental approach.* Help your client frame their change plan as an experiment, since this approach can reduce the pressure of feeling they must "succeed or fail" and it allows them to learn from the experience. We often say to our clients, "We're not the diet [or whatever behavior] police, but we're here to help you find what works for you, and we will keep working together until we find it." It's a good idea to remind clients about the spiral nature of change (Chapter 10) and normalize minor temporary lapses and restarts as part of the experiential learning journey.

4. *Listen for signs of readiness and proceed only when the client is ready.* As we said earlier, you can check for readiness by offering a recapitulation of the change talk you heard and then follow up with a key question to evoke what the client will *do* now that they are on the far side of the MI hill. This is not asking for commitment but offering space to consider possibilities and choices for moving forward.

Specific Steps for Developing a Plan

Below is a list of some specific steps you might use when assisting in the planning task.

1. *First listen for mobilizing change talk.* The first and most important skill is to listen for mobilizing language and determine the client's willingness and ability to take the next step. Any forward momentum in the form of a specific intention to act is a good sign that change will likely happen (Gollwitzer, 1999). When you hear words and phrases such as "possibly," "I could consider," "thinking on it," or "I might try," these indicate movement toward commitment, and you recognize you are on the mobilizing side of the MI Hill. It's unnecessary to wait—or push—for stronger language such as "I definitely will," since doing so could halt the progress.

2. *Evoke the next steps; evoke hope and confidence.* As mentioned, you can summarize the change talk and then ask a key open question that elicits possible ways to move forward. In planning, it's helpful to know how *confident* clients are that they can do what they intend. Recall that using the scaling questions can evoke more confidence if needed (Chapter 10).

3. *Respond to confidence talk.* When you hear people voicing positive arguments for why and how change can happen and their perceived ability

to succeed, use the OARS skills directionally to shine a light on the confidence talk and respond in a way to strengthen it.

- Questions ask for *elaboration* or examples of confidence talk.
- Affirmations highlight the person's capabilities, skills, and strengths.
- Reflections strategically target the commitment, change, or confidence talk.
- Summaries collect the person's voiced optimism about change.

4. *Identify and affirm strengths.* People can often adopt a skewed view of themselves and see only the negative first or overlook the inner resources and strengths already available to them. As discussed in Chapter 10, acknowledging and affirming strengths can boost low confidence. Although you can and should affirm, it is also effective to encourage clients to personally articulate these strengths and discover how they manifest in their daily lives. Naturally, the conversation will also explore how clients can leverage these strengths to their advantage in the present circumstances.

5. *Ask about past efforts and review past successes.* Inquiring about your clients' past efforts helps clarify their involvement in the planning task and prevents you from proposing something they have already attempted. People can identify their personal skills or strengths used in past successful situations—in a general sense—and apply them to their current situation.

6. *Create a list of possible choices.* Consider using the path-finding tool (Chapter 5) or something similar to assist your clients in mapping out various possibilities for reaching their goals. Many clients appreciate seeing all their possible next steps, and they refer to this as "brain dumping," which they say reduces the feeling of being overwhelmed or confused.

7. *Narrow down the list.* Once you have generated a list of ways to move forward, narrow it down and ask the client where they would like to begin—for example, "Based on what you know about yourself, which option would be a good starting point?"

8. *Brainstorm.* If your clients seem stuck, you can offer to brainstorm and, if needed, contribute your expertise and ideas (with permission) along with theirs. Stay in the coach approach and don your CAPE. Although you do not have *the* answers, your offerings will likely inspire your clients' creativity. Remember to refrain from giving personal comments on each idea and, instead, let the process happen swiftly to invite a robust list of options.

9. *Co-design.* Planning is a negotiation process, and you partner with clients to create personalized plans based on their preferences and needs. Guide the client in developing clear next steps, including what, when, how, and why. The SMART acronym (specific, measurable, attainable, realistic, and time bound) used in goal setting can help ensure success, and it can prompt you and your clients to consider specific details, define

measurements of success, create an achievable plan, and set a time frame for completion.

10. *Be mindful of the client's comfort level.* The way you conduct yourself can safeguard this planning task from being too overwhelming or too expansive in scope. Help a client break down the long- or mid-range goals into simple first steps and notice their level of comfort with the plan.

11. *Promote accountability.* Accountability goes deeper than merely checking in with the coach. The end objective is for people to take full responsibility for their actions, but it may require some time to acquire new habits or embark on new plans. You can provide the support needed in the early phases. In planning, you may ask clients how they will stay on track or how they would like to be accountable to themselves. Accountability is part of the structure provided in the coaching relationship and is the cornerstone of coaching.

12. *Strengthen the possibility of success.* Invite clients to consider resources, support, and potential obstacles as they create a plan. A collaborative relationship continues as you negotiate—not mandate—a plan. Beyond the initial plan, adjustments can be made for more frequent check-ins later, since ambivalence can return and interests wane. While stalls and restarts are common, you can help clients prepare for and recover from these. The planning task includes a discussion of and possible solutions for obstacles and setbacks and is an opportunity to evoke more commitment talk: "How will you stay on track?" "What support do you need?" (Expanding the various support resources can lessen the dependence on you, the coach.)

13. *Celebrate, acknowledge, and affirm small successes.* Invite clients to verbalize the positive arguments for change out loud, and to identify the possible ways they could celebrate progress and small successes. It's good for you to notice these successes, but even more important for the clients to express what they have learned about themselves and how they are succeeding.

MI USED THROUGHOUT THE SESSION

A common misconception is that MI is no longer needed once clients resolve their ambivalence, and their motivations seem solid. Perhaps evoking is not necessary (or advisable) if clients are ready for planning. However, other components of MI are still called for as much in planning as they were in the engaging, focusing, and evoking tasks. Planning is much more than ticking off a checklist of tasks to complete before the next session. The CAPE helps you set the guardrails of the session while clients experiment and consider the particulars of their own change plan. Partnership is needed, especially in the planning phase, as clients may face remaining goal confusion, ambivalence, or discrepancy. Acceptance and compassion provide the necessary support as clients embark on a novel and unfamiliar course of action.

Planning can be a joyful experience for you and your clients as they move forward toward their change goals. As fulfilling as it can be, it is also time to stay alert for certain pitfalls.

Planning Too Soon

If your clients do not seem ready to plan, pushing will not help. Ambivalence may reappear if the plan is premature or is not entirely theirs, and if you push, you can undo the progress made in engaging, focusing, and evoking.

A 2003 study (Amrhein et al., 2003) showed that in clients who had increasing commitment talk in MI sessions, two-thirds stopped their harmful drug use, and another third reduced it by half. But the no-change group also showed the same climb (with a few fluctuations) in their commitment language during the session. Then, surprisingly, there was a sharp decrease in commitment language at the end, and this group had no subsequent change in drug use. (See Figure 13.2.)

Miller and Rollnick (2002) posed an explanation for this dramatic difference. In the Amrhein study, the instructions asked therapists to follow a manual and develop a change plan with the clients at the end of the session. Although both groups showed increasing commitment language when therapists used MI, the no-change group had a sharp decrease in commitment language at the end when it was time for a change plan. These clients were apparently not ready to commit to a change plan, but the therapist manual directed them to get a plan anyway—and the result is that their commitment level fell back to zero. The therapists dutifully followed the manual and forged ahead to get a specific plan, regardless of the client's readiness. These therapists were, in essence, overlooking the signs presented to them by the clients and instead following the manual's instructions.

MI-consistent coaching is not about following a sequence of steps to "get the client to planning," but instead it invites you to listen and respond to the signs of readiness and adjust your coaching accordingly.

Coaching Sample: Planning Too Soon

Karen, a middle-school principal, came to coaching with a plan from her doctor. It read, "Begin a 21-day Elimination Diet, and avoid alcohol, sugar, gluten, dairy, and all forms of bread and pasta." Karen phoned to tell me (C. H. L.) she would start immediately. In fact, she had already removed the banned foods from her fridge and pantry and warned her spouse that

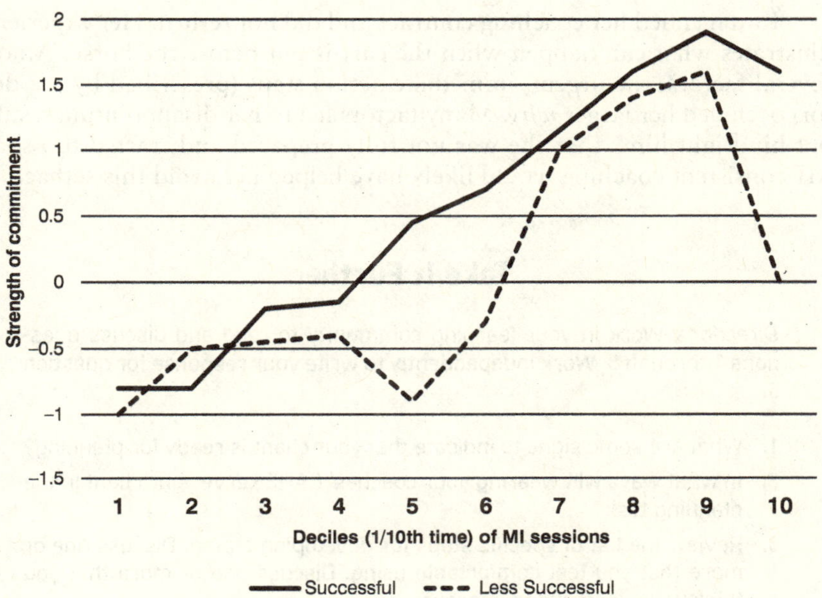

FIGURE 13.2. Strength of commitment language during MI sessions for clients with successful and less successful outcomes. Negative values represent commitment to continue drug use; positive values represent commitment to stop drug use. Data from Amrhein et al. (2003).

meals would be different for the next 3 weeks. Her long-term goal was to eventually transition from the Elimination Diet to one designed to help her lose the extra 100 pounds threatening her health. Despite her doctor's advice to see a coach before starting the diet, she began 1 week before our first visit. Her agenda for the first session included honing the details of the plan, brainstorming ideas for meal prep, and finding ways to avoid snacking in the workroom. But Karen experienced a significant setback between the first and second visits. Here is an account of the follow-up visit.

COACH: What were your wins from last week?

CLIENT: I didn't have any! I failed miserably. The stress at work is very high. I didn't have time to eat before the afternoon board meeting, so I dropped into the workroom and ate a bagel with cream cheese. Afterward, I felt so guilty about it that I started crying. I'm a grown woman, crying about eating a bagel! I left the board meeting as soon as it was over and went home, crying all the way. I felt so awful about it that I drank a whole bottle of wine and ate an entire pizza and an order of brownies. I got off my diet and haven't been able to start again.

Karen ended her coaching contract and did not return. Her experience illustrates what can happen when the cart is put before the horse. Among several factors, the urgent, immediate action steps (prescribed by the doctor) occluded her larger *why*. Many factors led to her disappointing results, but hindsight hints that she was not fully prepared and started too soon. MI-consistent coaching would likely have helped her avoid this setback.

Take It Further

Directions: Work in your learning community to read and discuss questions 1 through 5. Work independently to write your response for question 5.

1. What are some signs to indicate that your client is ready for planning?
2. In what ways will wearing your coaches' CAPE serve your client in the planning task?
3. Review the list of specific steps for developing a plan. Discuss one or more that you feel comfortable using. Discuss one or more that you think you would like to improve.
4. As a coach, how can you maintain calm restraint when you feel a sense of urgency to speed up the planning task for your client? What strategies can you use in such situations?
5. What are some ways to test the way to see if your client is ready to plan?

Part III

Building Skill and Improving Motivational Interviewing in Coaching

To aid you in applying the various MI theories and methods in your coaching practice, we offer a bird's eye view of how the individual pieces might fit together as a whole and then zoom in to suggest specific ways to examine and improve your practice.

MI is a research-based, effective method for facilitating your clients' change and growth. Chapter 14 presents practical ways to seamlessly weave those evidence-based theories and strategies in a coaching session. The four tasks (engaging, focusing, evoking, and planning) fit hand in glove with the structure and arc of the coaching process.

Chapter 15 answers, "How can I build and improve MI-consistent coaching?" Learning styles vary, but to improve, most of us need to review, examine, experiment, and intentionally apply knowledge into practice. We draw on our experience as educators, learners, coach trainers, and practitioners of MI-style coaching to provide practical ways for improving. However, these are not the only ways. We hope Chapter 15 serves as a starting point for exploring more ways to build and improve your coaching with MI.

Chapter 14

Putting It All Together

So far, we have written about the foundational spirit of MI (the coaches' CAPE), the four tasks, and the four core skills. We examined each component separately, and in this chapter, we reassemble them together into a whole. Looking separately at each element may leave the impression that coaching with MI follows a prescribed script and a rigid order. In fact, MI is a dynamic conversation, much like a dance, where you remain flexible and adjust to the needs of your client in the moment. Still, there is a general sequence of tasks within which you will use any combination of core skills and, throughout each session, continue to embrace the MI spirit. This chapter provides an overview of this sequence to answer questions about where you might use the skills and how they relate to the four tasks and the spirit of MI.

RECAP OF MI SPIRIT AND THE COACHES' CAPE

By now, you know MI is rooted in certain beliefs and assumptions about people. In summary, you work as a partner with people who are experts in their own lives, who have their own inner motivations and can find their own solutions. You evoke what is already there; you do not inject something that is missing. In this goal-oriented style, you explore a person's ambivalence and then the possibilities and plans for growth in an atmosphere of compassion and acceptance.

How is this accomplished? Throughout this book, the recurrent theme is that you guide rather than simply follow or lead. You may move in either direction on a continuum between following or leading, but generally, MI lands in the middle, with guiding. A central point of MI is that you can arrange the conversation and do something to influence your client within the coaching relationship and, specifically, within the coaching conversation. You use MI skills to facilitate forward movement, but the *way* you use the skills makes the difference. MI is much more than a list of skills and strategies; it begins with a heart and mindset.

This heart and mindset, the MI spirit, what we call the coaches' CAPE, answers two major questions: "Why should I want to learn the MI spirit?" and "How will I use the MI spirit in my practice?" You want to learn it because, without it, MI could become a complex technique and begin to feel like a lot of work, which can be tiresome. But with it, you can witness empowered people searching for and choosing change for their own reasons. There is great fulfillment in witnessing people explore and grow rather than trying to persuade or fix them. Wearing the coaches' CAPE is a reminder of the foundational mindset that influences the *way* you do everything else you do.

In previous discussions, we referred to both the MI spirit and the coaches' CAPE. In this chapter, we will mainly use the acronym CAPE as a helpful way to remember the four essential components that embody the essence of MI-consistent coaching. Below is a refresher on the coaches' CAPE. Later, we provide a blueprint of the four tasks viewed as a whole, how the CAPE is applied, and then look at each individual task. We include in Handout 14.1 (available online at *www.guilford.com/lanier-materials*) a bulleted list of the essence of each task, what you might *do* (the skills), and who you are *being* (spirit) in the task.

The Coaches' CAPE

Compassion—Not sympathy or pity but a conscious effort to prioritize your clients' needs and actively work toward their well-being. It is the foundation of a trusting relationship.

Acceptance—A deep appreciation for your clients and their perspectives. It includes accurate empathy, honoring autonomy, affirmations, and absolute worth.

Partnership—There are two experts in this relationship. You are the expert in coaching, and your clients are experts in their own lives.

Empowerment—MI is strengths-focused and assumes people already have their own genius, resources, motivations, and solutions. You work together to find it and call it forth.

STRUCTURE

Figure 14.1 is a reference for understanding the whole context of coaching with MI. It provides a snapshot representing a single coaching conversation and depicts both the framework and the directional flow of the session.

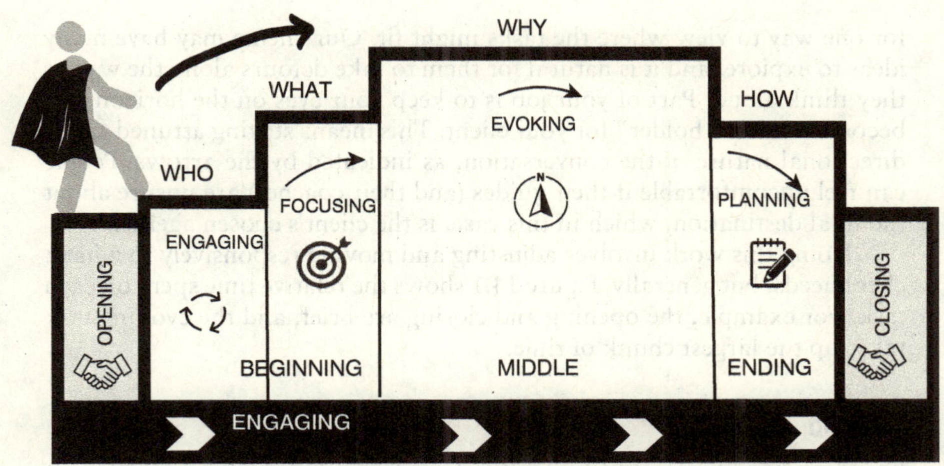

FIGURE 14.1. The four tasks of MI.

First, we explain it broadly, but later we zoom in on each task to help you orient where, when, and how you might incorporate the specific skills and spirit into each task. This snapshot reflects the general rhythm of the conversation. The client leads by choosing the agenda, and your job is to provide the structure of the conversation so that clients explore their reality, motivations, and potential choices and plans for moving forward. A coaching scenario is included to demonstrate the use of MI throughout a coaching conversation.

With the right heart and mindset, you enter the coaching session and work in a goal-oriented way within the four tasks. As previously stated, these tasks (engaging, focusing, evoking, and planning) are not strictly linear; you may cycle back to any of those tasks when clients need it. But generally, the tasks correlate to the beginning, middle, and end of coaching sessions. There is not one "right way" to do coaching, but the four tasks can provide guardrails to help you understand and gain mastery in conducting coaching conversations. As you gain experience coaching with MI, we encourage you to personalize your sessions to maintain engagement for both you and your client. Figure 14.1 (which we also presented at the introduction to Part II) suggests a general sequence for using MI skills and the coaches' CAPE from one task to the next.

THE FOUR TASKS OF MI: A BROAD VIEW

The four tasks can be thought of as falling in a sequence, with a beginning, middle, and end. We added opening and closing sections as bookends for one way to view where the tasks might fit. Our clients may have many ideas to explore, and it is natural for them to take detours along the way as they think aloud. Part of your job is to keep your eyes on the horizon and become a "vision holder" for your client. This means staying attuned to the directional nature of the conversation, as indicated by the arrows. People can feel uncomfortable if their guides (and their coaches) are unsure about the final destination, which in this case, is the client's chosen agenda.

Doing this work involves adjusting and moving responsively to what a client needs, but generally, Figure 14.1 shows the relative time spent on each task. For example, the opening and closing are brief, and the evoking task takes up the largest chunk of time.

Opening

Engaging begins here and builds the foundation for working together. It starts as you prepare before the meeting to be in a calm and present state. When you have a calm presence and pace your responses, clients are more likely to feel free to talk without being rushed. Good listening includes waiting for your client to respond, which invites them to become more active versus passive partners. One way to begin is to ask about wins from the previous week and respond with affirmations and convey hope. See the Opening section in Handout 14.1 for a quick reference on how the skills and the coaches' CAPE can be used throughout the session, starting with the opening.

The coaching excerpts below are examples of using MI throughout the coaching relationship, from the opening session onward. Jada wanted help to decide about her future. Specifically, she was choosing whether to pursue higher education or start a different career. She entered her "dream job" after high school, but after becoming disillusioned, she decided to move back home and explore other options. Although her case is presented as a threaded unit throughout this chapter, the following excerpts represent only portions from multiple sessions over time. Each excerpt pulls out one specific part of the four tasks, as well as the opening and closing. Jada came for 12 sessions over a period of 4 months. Although the opening is not one of the four tasks, we insert it here to show how the MI spirit and skills are used from the beginning to the end of each session. This first excerpt is taken from her third visit and shows the MI-consistent approach in the opening.

MI-Consistent Coaching in Opening

COACH: Hi, Jada! It's good to talk with you again. What's one thing you're pleased with since our last visit.	[*Warm welcome, engaging.*]

JADA: Last week was emotionally hard, but I'm better today. I'll be fine after this whole thing is behind me. Making big changes is hard, and I can get stressed, but today I've got a fresh start.

COACH: That sounds like a tough week. What makes today feel like a fresh start? [*Empathy, open question.*]

JADA: It was a hard decision to move home, but now I feel like I can start thinking about my future.

COACH: You've kept a positive outlook throughout this whole experience, even though that must have been challenging. [*Affirmations, reflective listening, and empathy.*]

JADA: Thanks. It was a hard but I'm hoping things get better.

Engaging

The opening serves as a brief welcome and opens the door for a more in-depth conversation. The engaging task is not distinct from the opening, but here, we look at them separately to suggest timing and the natural flow of things. As a review, engaging does not start and stop with each new task but is woven throughout your entire interaction. Notice in Figure 14.1 how engaging continues throughout all tasks.

Your client's success and retention hinge on the quality of your relationship with them; it's a deciding factor (Chapter 4). Engaging is different from the process of creating goals and is a time to focus on the *who* instead of the *what,* the person instead of the goal. Empathic listening helps unearth your clients' broader concerns and can offset any urge to fix the problem and create goals before establishing the relationship. Good reflective listening is fundamental in engaging because it's hard to build the rest of the session without it.

One way to promote engagement is first to explore desires, dreams, and visions of your client's ideal self and future related to their goals for change. To truly know someone, it's essential to understand their core values and goals. This understanding helps you recognize their viewpoint and inner frame of reference. Knowing what your clients value can be a key to finding their motivation. You can also broaden their perspective by exploring goals for several years ahead, or medium- and long-term goals. See the Engaging section in Handout 14.1 for a summary of the skills and how you might use the CAPE in the engaging task, and all four tasks.

We pick up with Jada on her second session, and the dialogue below is only a portion of that session. Engaging skills continue beyond the boundaries of this task, but this excerpt shows how the spirit and skills are used toward the beginning of the session in the engaging task. Here, Jada is invited to explore her larger values and strengths, and positive characteristics.

MI-Consistent Coaching in Engaging

COACH: Thanks for completing the characteristics of successful changers worksheet. What did you find out about your positive qualities? [*Acknowledge efforts and positive qualities.*]

JADA: That was fun. I circled fairness, forgiveness, perspective, honesty, and humility. That's a pretty accurate picture of who I am.

COACH: It confirmed what you already knew. [*Reflection.*]

JADA: It was on point, except for the perspective one. I sometimes have a good perspective on other people's problems, but when it comes to my problems, I can get lost and don't think things through.

COACH: Your good perspective helps others more than yourself. [*Reflection.*]

JADA: Yeah, for example, one of my coworkers would blame other people and I told her, "You should let it go. You're the one getting hurt and being upset. Just let it go."

COACH: That's a mature awareness, and I notice you're pretty honest with people, too [*Affirmation.*]

JADA: Yeah, I like to be honest, and I don't like lying. It makes me feel guilty, so I've learned to be up-front with people.

COACH: You have perspective about others and are up-front and tell the truth with people. How does that show up in your own life? [*Reflection, open question to invite more.*]

JADA: Maybe I'm too up-front and can be very hard on myself. Especially in work or school situations, I like to bring down the hammer, and it's easy to be frustrated with myself.

COACH: So, this honesty can lead to being tough on yourself. [*Reflection.*]

JADA: Yeah, I'm honest, and I want others to be honest with me. I hate when people sugarcoat things. I say, "Just tell me your feelings." [*Gathering more about her perspectives.*]

COACH: What else did you notice on that list? [*Open question.*]

JADA: Forgiveness is a big one for me. If people aren't kind to me, I continue being kind. I try to have people in my life who I can have deep connections and conversations with.

COACH: So, you forgive people even if they're not kind to you. What is most important to you? [*Reflection, open question (values).*]

JADA: I feel my career or just my general happiness in life is most important. There's more to life than just surface relationships.

COACH: You're good at knowing what matters in your life, like happiness, and getting to deeper things. [*Affirmation, reflection.*]

JADA: Thanks. I noticed this when I was younger. Now, I enjoy life more when I don't worry about those things.

COACH: You have a clear idea on what you want from life. What other strengths seem to describe you well? [*Affirmation, open question.*]

JADA: I need beauty; I'm an aesthetics person. For example, when I was young, I wouldn't go to a certain restaurant because it was ugly.

COACH: You have a pretty strong drive to be surrounded by something that appeals to you aesthetically. [*Reflection.*]

JADA: Yes! Being passionate about something drives me. I was pretty passionate about not going to that restaurant!

COACH: Passion helps you make choices about what's important to you. [*Reflection.*]

JADA: Yeah, but being passionate about something also causes me stress. I go back and forth in my head. I let things get to me easily and go to a negative mindset for a while. [*She begins to present her current dilemma.*]

COACH: So, there's a tipping point. [*Reflection.*]

JADA: Yeah, when I start having anxiety about something, that's when things change. I think about college, but don't know what to study and even though studying about people would be exciting, the thought of completing a lot of schoolwork stresses me out. [*A clue about what is important and what may be a focus.*]

COACH: Stress and anxiety seem to be roadblocks. [*Reflection.*]

JADA: Yeah, big ones.

COACH: Jada, you have a good perspective about other people, and you say you sometimes have trouble with perspective for yourself. You're pretty clear that having beauty and aesthetics are important to you and can even drive your decisions. When thinking about whether or not to go to school, you're concerned it could cause stress, and this makes the decision hard. What other things might be important for you to think about in our work together? [*Summary, highlight positives, empathic listening to understand the client, open question regarding the broad area of focus.*]

JADA: My biggest thing right now is deciding on college or a career. I'm very wishy-washy about this. I enjoy certain things, like analyzing people, but what do I do for the rest of my life? This is a big deal to me because I want to be happy and do what fits me most.

COACH: You know that whatever you choose has to fit you and be something you can be happy about. [*Reflection; not yet directional.*]

JADA: Right, and that's why I quit what was my perfect dream job. But here I am, no job. Now what? I guess I just don't know how to make the right decision. I hope you can help.	
COACH: I'm here to support you, and in the end, you get to make the choice. You've named some values already, and I have an activity that could help you find your most important core values. Does this interest you?	[*Partnership, honoring autonomy, sharing information with permission (A-O-A).*]
JADA: That's definitely something I'd love. I'm interested in those things and analyzing what makes people tick, including me.	[*Transition to focusing.*]

Focusing

With a trusting relationship built, the second task is finding a focus for the conversation. Without a clear focus, you could follow the conversation in wandering tangents. A collaborative approach can help negotiate the topic of your conversation, which may come from a straightforward question such as, "What do you want to work on today?" The answer may be clear, but at other times, several topics emerge, or there are many paths to take toward one goal. For these times, the path-finding tool (Chapter 5) is one way to organize the options visually. Pausing to step outside the conversation might give you and your client time to consider the way ahead. This pause is well worth the time, since you achieve very little in the evoking and focusing tasks without a clear focus. Remember, this is a goal-oriented conversation, but the agenda involves more than a list of change goals; it encompasses peoples' hopes, fears, expectations, and concerns.

The focus of the session can be twofold. There is an immediate goal for the individual session and a larger, mid- or long-range goal for 3 to 6 months in the future. An even broader view of the horizon can connect the dots between the vision and the goals and become a motivator. The search for a focus may involve orienting the client toward the larger horizon. See the Focusing section in Handout 14.1 for how you can use the MI skills and the coaches' CAPE in the focusing task.

The dialogue below is extracted from Jada's sixth session and shows the CAPE and skills used in the focusing task. It includes a midpoint check-in on goals. Engaging continues, and you may also find that evoking is needed at times.

MI-Consistent Coaching in Focusing

COACH: You created a powerful vision in the first session and then set a 3-month goal to decide between college or a career. Is this a goal that you want to keep working toward? [*Goal check-in.*]

JADA: Yeah, that still sounds good to me.

COACH: You took several steps already; in fact, you took a huge step to quit a job that didn't fit you. [*Affirmation.*]

JADA: Thanks. I debated whether I did the right thing.

COACH: You also mentioned that you might want to work on having a better headspace to have more peace and not stress so much while making this decision. [*Affirm efforts, empowerment.*]

JADA: Yeah, I think this negative headspace is a problem, like when I feel wrong because I'm different than a lot of people I know. It sort of keeps me stuck.

COACH: Tell me more about what you want, that vision of Jada you described at the beginning of our work together. [*Connects goal with a broader vision.*]

JADA: My vision includes a career that brings happiness and fulfillment, one I'm passionate about. I want to enjoy the moments and not worry about the future so much. I want perspective and self-understanding, and it would be nice to have hope right about now. I need to be inspired and connected with people who are like me, people who aren't just getting through life.

COACH: A positive headspace brings you closer to the happiness and fulfillment you want. And hope will help, too. [*Reflection (a guess).*]

JADA: Yeah, hope is a lot more "flowy" than a plan. There's a lot of pressure with a plan, but I guess a plan keeps you on track. [*Clues about how she prefers to work.*]

COACH: So, you'd rather have something more inspiring and hopeful instead of a plan that makes you feel pressured. [*Reflection.*]

JADA: Right. My negative thoughts get in the way. I hold myself back a lot just thinking about what could go wrong, so I want to get out of that headspace. I want to try things, like looking at different careers or visiting some colleges. But I think about how I could fail and cycle those thoughts instead of enjoying things. Negative thinking also hurts my relationships, and we might work on that.

COACH: What things have worked for you in the past to get out of that headspace? [*Evoking woven in with focusing, reflection.*]

JADA: Movement, going to the gym, and listening to music. Those work, at least for a little bit.

COACH: You want to find ways to get out of your negative headspace, make plans to visit colleges, or learn about different jobs, and maybe work on relationships. Which feels like a good place to begin? [*Summary, partners to help narrow the focus.*]

JADA: I honestly don't know where to begin.

COACH: Here's a tool we could use to organize all your ideas and help you decide where to start. I can write down the ideas you've named, and we can add more if you need. [Coach writes choices on path-finder tool.]

COACH: (*After the activity.*) Which of these sounds more important as a place to start?

JADA: It makes sense to work on the headspace, don't you think? That'll help with being positive, more excited, and open to learning. Eventually, I need specific steps to decide between a career or college, but nothing that puts pressure on me. [*The client is tentative about a "plan."*]

COACH: We can work on the positive headspace first, and then if we have time, we could move to something else. How's that? [*Partnership, to narrow the focus.*]

JADA: That sounds like a good idea. Having more positive thoughts would help. Like I said, more excitement and more openness to learning. Those negative thoughts block me; for example, I'm losing skills like my art technique because I've stopped doing that. I guess I need some tools and maybe some ideas.

COACH: You've named a few things, like movement, drawing, and listening to music. I can offer a few things that others have used to help with a positive mindset. [*Reflection, partnership.*]

JADA: I definitely need that. Stress is a real problem, and when I think of the job I had, it's very stressful and scary.

An opening and engaging period preceded this focusing part of the session. Notice how the CAPE is used to help negotiate the focus of the conversation. In MI-consistent coaching, focusing means clarifying the specific topic of the session before moving on to why and how a person might make the change.

In Jada's case, the overall goal is clear, but the path to reaching it is unclear. Before heading out toward the evoking and planning phase, it's important to ensure that there is a clear, agreed-upon end target for the session. It's easy and natural for clients to wander around a topic for a while, and if this happens, you can put guardrails in place and gently guide the conversation back to the focus. You keep the conversation moving in the direction of your client's goals unless they choose a new one.

Jada's goal was expressed as *being* rather than *doing* (thinking positively vs. negatively), and it's harder to frame "thinking" into a specific action step. Still, as the focusing task unfolds, she and the coach gain more clarity about what she wants from the session. Your sessions do not always have to end with a "SMART" behavior change goal since coaching also fosters growth in perspective, insight, and learning. In this focusing task, the coach helps Jada choose from several possible paths to reach her goal of a "better headspace." We continue Jada's journey in the next task of evoking.

Evoking

The evoking task usually occurs in the middle of the session, after engaging and focusing, although evoking skills continue throughout the planning task. In the natural flow of conversations about change, you hear both change talk and sustain talk as a normal expression of ambivalence. (See "The MI Hill" in Chapter 6 as a review.)

In the evoking task, when you hear and recognize change talk among a mix of change talk and sustain talk, you invite clients to offer more change talk, and you strategically favor change talk and soften the sustain talk. Using the OARS skills tells you what to *do;* wearing the coaches' CAPE tells you the *way* to do it. You use the OARS skills in a directional way to elicit and strengthen a person's arguments for change so that they talk themselves into changing. Evoking may include the skill of providing information in the A-O-A format (Chapter 8) or using importance and confidence rulers as we discussed in Chapter 7. In Figure 14.1, note the arrow and compass in the evoking task, which suggest forward movement toward a client's true north, their aspirations, and goals for the future. See the Evoking section in Handout 14.1 for how you can use the MI skills and the CAPE in the evoking task.

Here is Jada's seventh session, with the portion that demonstrates the evoking task. Jada's focus for this session was finding ways to get in a better mindset so she could make decisions about her future. Evoking is easier to identify when there is clear ambivalence around a behavior change, such as quitting smoking. However, even when the topic is broader, as in this example, you can still use evoking skills to help the client move forward.

MI-Consistent Coaching in Evoking

COACH: You said you want freedom, flow, and new thinking, and yet you struggle with negative thinking. How did the negative headspace impact your work this week?	[*Reflect discrepancy, open question explores values.*]
JADA: I looked into physical therapy and felt it would suit me, but I started stressing out about the education and training. Part of me wants an art career, but other people say, "You won't make money, and you'll be unemployed," and then I get stuck and very stressed.	
COACH: What might happen if you don't get past this negative thinking?	[*Invite change talk, imagining extremes.*]

JADA: I might do what other people want but be unhappy with my life. Physical therapy would be the safe route, but would I look back and wonder if I should have gone for art? Did I settle? I'm not giving up on an art-related career, because I *need* color, beauty, and interesting things. Having a positive attitude would help me stay peaceful, so I can grow. I'm just stuck.

COACH: You want an attitude that allows you to grow. [*Reflect change talk.*]

JADA: Right. Instead of thinking about what could go right, I think about how I could fail and how I'm not qualified. I'm so focused on the future that I'm not growing right now. My art skills are lost.

COACH: You're stuck by cycles of negative thinking, and you want to be positive so you can grow and learn. [*Reflection (double-sided) with* and.]

JADA: Yes, I want to listen to people, but not be stressed by that so much that it stops my positive thinking. People think I should do logical jobs, like engineering, but that's stressful because I don't do those things well.

COACH: You know yourself best. You want to think in more positive ways and consider what's best for you. [*Affirm, directional reflection.*]

JADA: I do, but I beat myself up. It's just not how my brain works, and it's not fair! It seems so easy for everyone. I feel discouraged.

COACH: This is an example of the negative headspace. What kind of thinking would you need to help you move to a place of positivity? [*Directional open question.*]

JADA: I'm not sure. There's probably a different way to see it, but it's been ingrained in my head since I was young. People made jokes about that and it hurts my feelings.

COACH: You still remember what people said about you, and you think there's a different way to see things now. [*Reflecting ambivalence.*]

JADA: I would love to see it the other way, but it's difficult when people tell me otherwise. I can start believing in myself, but something happens. I'm afraid it'll be the same thing.

COACH: What are those beliefs you could have? [*Inviting change talk, exploring values.*]

JADA: I always fear I'm not going to be good enough. I want to believe that what I like and need are important.

COACH: What things do you like and need that are important to consider in this situation? [*Open, evoking question.*]

JADA: I like colorful, cool, interesting things and people with different perspectives on life. I want a schedule but not one that puts too much pressure on me, and I don't want to sit in a boring office staring at a white piece of paper and a computer. I want to be with friends and people like me and have more fun. I can imagine going out to some cool place for dinner or a coffee shop and doing simple, inspiring things. It doesn't have to be anything big, but not the same thing like a job I don't like for 40 years. I want to think differently and be inspired.

COACH: I notice a bit more positive shift in your mood when you name all those things. You say it brings comfort when you talk about the inspiring people, things, and color you want in your life. You seem to come to life when you describe that inspiring environment. I'm curious, what do you think would be the best outcome from having—and keeping—a positive mindset? [*Summary of change talk, open evoking question.*]

JADA: I would have the confidence to say, "This is what I'm good at, what I like, and what I've decided to do." I wouldn't worry what other people think.

COACH: Given where you are now with your mindset, how confident are you if 10 is "I'm very able to decide what I want to do" and 0 is "I'm not at all sure I can do this." [*A scaling question to evoke confidence.*]

JADA: Well, my mindset is still pretty bad, so my confidence is low, probably a 5.

COACH: Why a 5 and not a 2? [*Evoking confidence.*]

JADA: Well, I was brave enough to admit what I need and want in life. I already quit a job that didn't fit my values, so that's good. My mindset is at the place where I could shadow a local artist this week at our community art center. There are lots of interesting people there, and I would be inspired. That would be a good step. [*Imagining possibilities.*]

COACH: You're very good at self-awareness to want alignment with your values and what's important to you. [*Affirmation.*]

JADA: Thanks, I just need to stop placing all the stress on myself to be something I'm not. I want to feel free to be who I am, and accept myself. I could start drawing some and not be so critical. [*Change talk, and the beginning of activation to plan.*]

Planning

At some point in the evoking task, you may hear change talk that increases in frequency and strength, and you sense it's time to move forward. As we said in Chapter 13, you can test the water by asking a key question, such as "What do you think you'll do?" Or you could offer a summary first, followed by a key question about what your client might want to do next. If you hear mobilizing change talk in response, it might be time to transition to planning. But if there is more sustain talk, this may mean more time is needed for evoking.

After the uphill climb to prepare for change, you begin to travel downhill on the mobilizing side, which is about movement and action. Once it seems like it's time to begin planning (Chapter 13), your questions invite the client to make activation statements about a change. You may hear tentative language, such as "I might," "I could," or "I'd be willing to." These early statements might become firm commitments toward the end, but pushing for a commitment too soon might seem pushy and result in hesitancy or more sustain talk. After you have a change plan, a good strategy is to summarize and then ask about commitment.

Coaching creates movement partly because it implies accountability from clients to coaches and, more importantly, to themselves. Planning may end with open questions such as "What will you do," "By when?" "How will you know you have been successful?" or "How will you or others recognize success?" Self-monitoring is a way to strengthen commitment, and this takes many forms, such as journals, trackers, apps, and checklists. Part of the power of these strategies is that clients raise awareness of their ongoing behavior, thoughts, and decisions. MI skills can be used to evoke and explore the client's own ideas in this process.

The important thing to remember in planning is that the change plan is a negotiation. Planning is a genuine collaboration between you and the client, and this is when you restrain from delivering your expertise. Rushing this process can spoil a good coaching session.

As we said, there are situations where your clients' learning can be supplemented by providing additional information and advice, and this is compatible with MI as long as it respects people's freedom of choice. Use the A-O-A framework to provide support while also respecting clients' autonomy. The most important consideration is collaboration and agreement about what will happen next.

Sometimes, a good plan is just the next step for the client, not every step of the goal. The change plan can be a simple behavior or strategy the client creates. But sometimes, reaching a mid- or long-range goal can be a more complex series of steps. At times, we come across clients who may not be prepared for a comprehensive plan with detailed action steps. Instead, a first step may be researching, journaling, or having discussions about the specifics of how the plan would progress. All such "goals" are positive signs of movement forward and deserve to be acknowledged and celebrated. See the Planning section in Handout 14.1 for a summary of the skills and how you might use the CAPE in the planning task.

This excerpt picks up Jada's sixth session from the previous example in evoking. The first statement from the coach is a transition to planning based on the mobilizing change talk expressed previously.

MI-Consistent Coaching in Planning

COACH: You've been exploring how a positive headspace can help you better decide about going to college or starting a job. You said the headspace can help	[*Summary, followed by a key question.*]

you feel free to be who you are and flourish in a life that includes art and the inspirational things you need. What might you be considering at this point?

JADA: I could shadow an artist around here, but only if I'm ready. [*Tentative change talk.*]

COACH: Something might come before that step. [*Complex reflection.*]

JADA: I feel like I'm forcing it. Shadowing artists sounds like a plan, but it puts pressure on me, and I don't need that right now.

COACH: What else are you thinking might help? [*Evoking ideas.*]

JADA: I've journaled before, and that helps sometimes, but I lost some writing skills while working. A journal could be a good way to see what I'm thinking, if I don't focus on the negative. [*The client considers possible solutions with reluctance.*]

COACH: You can see the advantages and disadvantages. What other concerns might you have about this particular strategy? [*Reflection, exploring reluctance.*]

JADA: At my last job, I wrote about conforming to a different way of thinking. That was stressful, but identifying what was bothering me felt better. I want the freedom to be who I am, and I need to accept how my brain works and not be so hard on myself. I could start journaling or drawing and not be so critical about what I draw. Or maybe I can go into the city. It's a creative place and I could take a friend to visit museums or old churches and look at stained glass windows. [*Some commitment language ("I could," "I can").*]

COACH: You've had a sudden burst of insight! There's the creativity you mentioned before, and it shows up in the fun possibilities you're considering. Earlier, you said you have a good perspective for [*Affirmation and linking reflection.*]

others, and I see you have a pretty clear perspective about yourself, too.

JADA: Thanks. I think I'm happiest when I'm creative and inspired.

COACH: Which of those things you mentioned sound feasible now? *[Evoking action.]*

JADA: Journaling for sure. I think it would give me perspective and more self-understanding, and some hope for the future.

COACH: Earlier, you said you wanted a "flowy" hope, and that was different from a plan. How does this move you closer to flowy hope? *[Linking reflection, evoking action.]*

JADA: If I have a plan, that brings hope. But what if that plan messes up? Then you deviate after you've invested all this just to find out that it's not something you want. That's scary. *[Low confidence.]*

COACH: You don't want to feel disappointed if your plans don't work out. What would it be like to get past that scary feeling? *[Reflect meaning, evoking confidence.]*

JADA: It'd feel great! I think I'm already less scared because I came up with lots of creative things to do. Just breaking out of a stressful job is a good beginning. I'm definitely going to write in my journal and consider calling a friend and planning a trip to the city. *[Stronger commitment language.]*

COACH: Did you want to plan specifically for your visit to the city? *[Closed question used appropriately in negotiating the plan.]*

JADA: I may do that, but I need to build up to that first. Journaling is probably all I want to plan for this week.

COACH: You know what's best for you, and it's your choice. When might you want to start the journal? *[Affirm autonomy, ask for specifics.]*

JADA: I've already got a journal, so I can start in the morning.

COACH: What specifically might you want to commit to this week? [*Strengthen commitment.*]

JADA: I keep my journal by my desk, and every morning when I get my coffee I could sit down and write. I'll get my drawing and painting supplies down, too!

COACH: What might help you stay on track with your plan? [*Accountability.*]

JADA: I set reminders on my phone and usually follow through once I see that notification. I'll set the reminder for wake-up time.

COACH: What other support would you need to get this done? [*Support.*]

JADA: I don't have anyone else that I want to include. I think just coming back to see you next week is the only support I need.

COACH: Sounds good. How will you know you've been successful in using your journal to shift your mindset? [*Measures of success.*]

JADA: I'll be able to tell if my mood and headspace are better, and who knows, I might feel so positive that I call a few artists this week.

COACH: What kinds of obstacles could get in the way? [*Navigating obstacles.*]

JADA: Nothing, really. I've got what I need, and I can make this part of my daily routine.

Planning is the time to hold fast to the CAPE and remember the mindset of deeply trusting and respecting people's own solutions. Resist the temptation to fix the client and tell or persuade with your own experience or expertise. The planning task maintains the core spirit and skills of MI that you used in the previous tasks of engaging, focusing, and evoking. The same skills used in evoking are employed here to help strengthen the commitment to a change plan. Negotiating a change plan is not a final step but a beginning one.

Closing

The closing is both a gentle exit to the session and a commencement for the real work of change to come. Summarizing the plan and then expressing your belief and confidence in your client's abilities and strengths is a good way to close the session. You negotiated a feasible and personalized plan, but life has a way of dulling the edges of motivation in the space between sessions. The action stage of change is often the most challenging, so if your client reaches out, perhaps with written messages between visits, your MI coaching skills can shine through even in your responses. The advantage is that you can take time to choose your words carefully. You might need to affirm their efforts, help them refocus, provide some information, or assist them to adjust the plan as needed.

The session closing could include circling back to the original agenda to see if the client got what they needed from the session. If new topics arise, you can note these for follow-up sessions. See the Closing section in Handout 14.1 for a summary of the skills and how you might use the CAPE in the closing.

We proceed with Jada's sixth session and demonstrate how the CAPE and skills persist until the end. Like the opening, the closing is not distinct from the task before it but transitions naturally from planning. We separate it here to show how MI can be used to close the session.

MI-Consistent Coaching in Closing

COACH: Jada, you started with a goal to find ways to get into a better headspace so you can make decisions about your future. The first step is to write your thoughts in your journal, and you're even going to try to draw again. Thanks for being honest to talk about what you need, and then working on a plan. What is one of your major learnings from today?	[*Summary, affirmation, and open question.*]
JADA: I'm learning that I put some limits on myself, and I'm slowly finding ways to get past those limits.	
COACH: From what you've told me, it sounds like you'll find those ways. Does this feel like a good time to wrap up our session today?	

JADA: Sure, I think it's good.

COACH: Did you get everything you needed in today's session?

JADA: Yes, maybe next time I can plan to visit some colleges.

COACH: We can definitely work on that next time. See you soon!

Jada's case offered many valuable coaching lessons. As a young woman in a major transition phase and searching for answers, she reminded us that people have their own wisdom and can indeed find their own solutions. It's a joy to witness people become empowered to uncover their inner genius, and MI-consistent coaching paved the way for this growth.

Early in our sessions, there were tears as Jada struggled to find peace. Over time, she became more empowered to stand up for what she felt was right for her. She used many tools to manage stress, such as journaling, meditating, and finding ways to calm and quiet the internal saboteur that put her down. After a few weeks, her confidence was growing: "I think there are options for me, and no matter what I do, if I give it my best, that's all I can do." By the end of our sessions, she had the consistent "positive headspace" she was looking for.

Jada's immediate steps were tied to her larger goal of making a choice for her future. The values of beauty, creativity, learning about human behavior, and having deep and interesting relationships were motivating forces drawing her forward. She longed for a life aligned with those values. Jada grew to accept her unique talents and characteristics, and she made choices for a future that would honor her true self.

After 3 months of our working together, Jada had not yet made a definite choice about the trajectory of her life. However, the quotes below—her responses to the question "What is your most significant insight from our session today?"—demonstrate the significant progress and personal development she gained through coaching.

"I've grown more than I thought."

"I'm proud of myself."

"It doesn't all have to be figured out right now, and that's good! That's where you can learn from your mistakes and live life the best you can."

Jada has now chosen to enter college and study nutrition. She enrolled in pottery and art classes and hopes to continue taking art classes throughout college.

Take It Further

Directions: Handout 14.1 (online at *www.guilford.com/lanier-materials*) presents the opening, engaging, focusing, evoking, planning, and closing sections of a coaching conversation. Work with your learning community and use the handout to help you answer the questions below.

1. Review the Opening section in Handout 14.1 and then create an opening statement that reflects the purpose and tone of the coaching session.
2. Review the Engaging section in Handout 14.1. What do the circular arrows suggest? What is your primary role in engaging, and how might this look different than in the evoking task?
3. Review the Focusing section in Handout 14.1. What are some important things for you, the coach, to remember in the focusing task? What components of the coaches' CAPE will be called for in the focusing task?
4. Review the Evoking section in Handout 14.1. How do the core skills (OARS) become directional in the evoking task? What is meant by "E" in CAPE, and how is this used in the evoking task?
5. Review the Planning section in Handout 14.1. How can each of the OARS skills be used to evoke in the planning task? What can you do if your client has low confidence in the planning task?
6. Review the Closing section in Handout 14.1. Create a closing statement using one of the skills.

Chapter 15

Learning and Improving Coaching with Motivational Interviewing

> I hear and I forget, I see and I remember,
> I do, and I understand.
>
> —CONFUCIUS

Reading this book and attending workshops lays an essential base of knowledge you can build on, but applying this knowledge and improving in practice requires more. To become proficient in any complex skill, it's usually necessary to observe your practice, review it, get specific feedback, then develop goals for improvement. Simply practicing may not lead to improvement in MI, but *guided* practice with feedback is the added component that can make a difference for most people. This is often called deliberate, targeted practice, and regardless of your prior background, you can improve your skills by engaging in this type of practice (Ambrose et al., 2010).

When a baseball player repeatedly hits a pop fly, it's easy for the opposing team to catch it, and it usually results in an out. The baseball coach advises the player to practice hitting, so the player enters the batting cages and begins to practice. However, automatic feedback from each swing confirms that no adjustments were made, and nothing changed. The player becomes even more proficient at hitting the pop fly ball rather than improving. Specific feedback from someone more skilled is needed to change the course and correct the mistake.

Specific feedback is fundamental for any learning, and real-time embedded feedback particular to the intended performance goal is the most helpful. Without feedback, learners can assume everything is fine, and they continue practicing in the same way. This leads to an inaccurate assessment of skills and abilities (Hardavella et al., 2017).

Extensive research verifies the efficacy of MI; however, as with any complex skill, the effectiveness of this method depends on practitioners' skill levels and their proficiency in using MI. A subjective feeling about how well you use MI is not the most accurate way to judge proficiency because most people have a much higher view of their skill than their practice indicates. But take heart; becoming proficient in coaching with MI is possible with practice over time. This chapter is a guide for getting there.

Chapter 14 focused on combining the various components of MI to form a cohesive and integrated system. This chapter offers methods to reflect upon and improve your MI skills in practice. (For a bulleted list of lessons learned from the research on learning and improving MI skills, see the document "Research on Coaching with Motivational Interviewing," available online at *www.guilford.com/lanier-materials*.)

To improve in a complex skill such as MI, a good plan is to focus on one goal at a time, practice thoroughly, reflect, and get feedback to assess how close you came to achieving the goal. The next step could be developing a personalized plan for growth and then starting the cycle again. Intentional reflection and feedback can help you measure your current skill level and pinpoint improvement areas. To get started, you might ask, "What should I observe?"; "What are some ways to get feedback on my practice?"; and "How do I know if I'm doing MI?"

Defining the standards that determine proficiency is essential when getting started. You can then use these criteria as benchmarks to assess your MI skill. Our intent in this chapter is to provide a concise and clear roadmap for improving your MI-consistent coaching practice. We provide tables, worksheets, bulleted lists, and handouts as convenient tools for observing, reflecting, offering and receiving feedback, and creating new goals for further improvement.

ASSESSING PROFICIENCY IN THE FOUR TASKS

What standards would you look for to assess proficiency in the four MI tasks? Focusing on the job at hand while actively listening to your client can be a tricky balancing act, but this is the art of professional coaching, and you can improve with intentional practice. Sometimes, you may feel lost in a session and wonder what is happening and where to go next. The point we made in Chapter 14 was that the four MI tasks of engaging, focusing, evoking, and planning can help you navigate the session and find your way.

The four tasks are layered and sequential, and you can move flexibly from one to the other. What you do in one task can impact another task. Evoking the possibilities of change may increase readiness to plan, and careful listening in focusing can boost client engagement needed in evoking. Even with these overlaps of the four tasks, it can be helpful to step back and see which tasks might need more emphasis.

With reflective listening, it is possible to assess during a session which task seems to need attention. Have you made progress in the engaging task? Do you have a clear agenda for the session? Have you heard change talk, and does the client seem ready to plan? These prompts can help you determine the progress you and your client have made in engaging, focusing, evoking, and planning tasks and adjust as needed.

It could be helpful to review the suggested questions in Table 15.1 before a session. Then, during a session, you might be able to gain perspective and decide if you want to steer the conversation in a specific direction. After a session, you can use these questions as a guide for self-reflection or peer feedback on what went well and what you would like to improve.

Not every session includes all four tasks, but if you collected data over one or more sessions, you could study the sequencing and depth of each task. You might want to create your own system to measure your proficiency; otherwise, the questions in Table 15.1 can be a helpful guide for reflecting on your use of the skills in each of the four tasks. The results can help you choose new learning goals. (The same questions are available in Handout 15.1 at *www.guilford.com/lanier-materials.*)

MEASURING CLIENT RESPONSES

The previous discussion is a guide for measuring your responses, but what about comments by the client? Listening to what clients say can indicate the extent to which your responses strengthen change talk and soften sustain talk, for example. As we said, more change talk predicts and facilitates positive change outcomes, and change talk is expected to rise over the course of an MI-consistent session. The ratio of change talk to sustain talk can indicate, among other things, your proficiency in increasing the client's change talk. A reasonably easy coding system for counting and measuring change talk or sustain talk is the Client Language Easy Rating (CLEAR), and you can find a link at *www.guilford.com/lanier-materials.*

In the future, you might employ a trained MITI (motivational interviewing treatment integrity) coder who will use that or a similar form to provide you with more specific feedback and even a narrative report. You can find MITI coders via a link at *www.guilford.com/lanier-materials.*

But for a start, we offer an even easier and more accessible method. This simplified method can help you track the frequency and amount of client change talk and your responses in a coaching session. Furthermore, you can see how your language influences your client's responses toward (or away from) the desired change or growth goal. It can be informative to

TABLE 15.1. Suggested Open Questions for Measuring Skill in the Four Tasks

Engaging

- Do I understand my client's perspectives on the situation or dilemma?
- Do I ask more open than closed questions?
- Do I talk less than half of the time?
- Do I change questions to reflections instead? (Drop the tone at the end.)
- Do I acknowledge and affirm my client's positive traits and efforts?
- Do I acknowledge specific things my client has done as well as their enduring and commendable qualities?
- Do I offer an equal number of reflections to questions? Do I offer twice as many reflections to questions?
- Do I use OARS without necessarily using them in a goal-directed way?
- Do I notice the client's level of engagement in our conversation?
- Do I use complex reflections more than simple reflections (rephrasing)?
- Do I use reframing as a complex reflection to offer a different meaning?
- Do I understand discord when I hear it, and do I know how to diffuse it?
- Do I gather together and summarize what the client said?

Focusing

- Do I help clients choose a clear agenda for the session?
- Do I help maintain the direction toward the agenda after the focus is clear?
- Do we have a working alliance toward agreed-upon goals?
- Do I help clients connect goals to their larger horizons, dreams, and values?
- Do I use a decisional balance to maintain neutrality if I feel it's necessary?

Evoking

- Do I know enough about this client's motivations for change?
- Do I recognize change talk (DARN CATS)? Do I intentionally respond to evoke and strengthen it?
- Do I use directional questions to cultivate change talk and ask for examples and elaboration?
- Do I recognize sustain talk and respond in a way to minimize rather than maximize it?
- Do I use OARS skills in a directional way, and respond to change talk when it happens?
- Do I know the client's ideas, goals, or values that would be motivators for change?
- Do I use affirmations, reflections, and summaries in a way to strengthen and ask for more change talk?
- Do I hear a shift to more change talk than sustain talk as a result of evoking?
- Do I use the ask–offer–ask method to provide information or advice?
- Do I plant seeds for change talk when there seems to be little of it?
- Do I gather change talk statements and offer them as a "bouquet" summary?

(continued)

TABLE 15.1. *(continued)*

Planning
• Do I check for client readiness to transition from evoking to planning? • Do I wait on my client's readiness and avoid planning prematurely? • Do I defer to my client's ideas for how to make a change? • Do I evoke mobilizing (CATs) change talk rather than trying to suggest or inject my solutions? • Do I empower my client to explore possible ways forward? • Do I use MI skills to strengthen my client's confidence if it seems to be low? • Do I facilitate my client's discovery of their strengths and past successes?

notice the volley of statements between you and your client and this may help you determine what adjustments you might want to make. What did you say in response to a client's change talk or sustain talk? What did you say prior to a client's change talk or sustain talk? Did you maximize change talk? Did you minimize sustain talk? You can count your reflections and questions and notice how your clients respond to them.

The tool for measuring change talk and sustain talk seen in Box 15.1 could measure your ability to evoke change talk, a primary aim of MI-consistent coaching. It could also be a way to attune your ear to the sounds of the language of change, both sustain talk and change talk. Remember, before inviting and strengthening change talk, you must first recognize what it sounds like. If you are just starting on this approach, it can be hard to hear the nuances of change talk in a session, and this tool allows you to become more conscious and aware of what to listen for in future practice.

Instead of trying to remember what happened in the conversation, recordings of your sessions provide a more accurate review and allow pausing, reversing, and fast-forwarding. When you go back and review your practice, you might be better able to notice things you missed during the session. You could use the recording for yourself as a postsession self-reflection tool. Or you might use the recording (with your client's written permission) with a mentor or with peer coaches within a professional learning community. Box 15.1 (also available online as Handout 15.2 at *www.guilford.com/lanier-materials*) is a breakdown of the straightforward approach.

MEASURING SPECIFIC SKILLS

To delve deeper, you might try measuring specific MI skills. The MITI tool offers detailed and tested definitions and rules for each specific behavior and for how they are counted (*www.motivationalinterviewing.org/sites/default/files/miti4_2.pdf*). But for a start, you can do this without using the

BOX 15.1. Tool for Measuring Change Talk and Sustain Talk

PURPOSE

Within a coaching conversation, you might hear signals that the client is moving toward the desired change. As this happens, one expects a higher percentage of change talk to sustain talk as the session unfolds. This shift is predictive of future change (or no change) and could provide indicators of your growing skill of evoking.

SETUP

- Get written consent from your client to record the session. Explain the policy for disposing of recordings after a specific time.
- Audio record a coaching session. While not required, consider an automated recording software that provides a written transcript of the recording. A simple internet search for accurate and economical programs will provide many choices.
- Make any edits to the transcript as needed and identify the speakers. (Some programs will automatically label speakers after you enter the names once or twice.)
- One option is to print out the transcript so you can "mark it" or color code as you listen. However, a Word document can also serve this purpose since there is a way to "mark" text with colors.

ACTIVITY

This simple system is a way to observe and visibly code the amount of change talk and sustain talk in a session. A first pass lets you identify and highlight the client's change talk and sustain talk. Afterward, you could review the session a second time to notice what you (or another coach) said that seemed to evoke change talk or soften sustain talk. As mentioned, you can use this to reflect on your own sessions or give feedback to others.

If you have a printed transcript, one option is to use a green highlighter to mark client change-talk statements and a yellow highlighter to mark client sustain-talk statements. This provides an immediate snapshot of the amount and ratio of change talk to sustain talk. If you prefer not to print the transcript, you could try the highlight text feature in a Word document to mark change talk green and sustain talk yellow.

(continued)

Step 1

1. Read the transcript of the coaching session.
2. Find the ***client*** statements that indicate movement toward the desired change (change talk). Use a green highlighter to mark these statements.
3. Find the ***client*** statements that indicate movement away from change or toward sustaining the target behavior (sustain talk). Use a yellow highlighter to mark these statements.

Step 2

1. Read the transcript a second time.
2. Find the ***coach*** statements and consider these questions.
   a. When change talk appeared, what happened just before it? After it?
   b. When sustain talk appeared, what happened just before it? After it?
   c. What seemed to evoke change talk? (Change talk is often mixed with sustain talk, and you may have to look closely to find it.)
   d. What did you do to maximize or minimize sustain talk?

Step 3

Review the session for proficiency. Now that you have a visible representation of your client's change talk and sustain talk and your responses before and after, what is the proficiency measurement? As we said, specialized tools are available to code change talk and sustain talk, but for starters, a simple count of change-talk and sustain-talk statements can be informative. You can also notice how much the ratio changes as the session unfolds. An equal frequency of change talk to sustain talk reflects ambivalence and predicts no change, but as the session continues, one hopes to see the balance shift to more change talk.

Here is one suggestion for reviewing the highlighted transcript to measure and plan for your growth in MI. As you would for those you coach, wear the strengths-colored lenses while you view your own (or others') transcripts. Remember to celebrate what went well and your progress so far, then choose one thing to target for further practice. We offer this as only one way to measure your skills of acknowledging, inviting, and strengthening change talk while minimizing sustain talk. You can look at several things in addition to what is listed below, and of course, consider developing other strategies that work for you.

1. Count the number of change-talk and sustain-talk statements.

2. How many change-talk statements are there compared to sustain-talk statements? How does this change throughout the session?

3. Consider a few things you did especially well and one specific area you would like to focus on for future practice and improvement. You may have noticed the ability to soften sustain talk effectively. Maybe your affirmations evoked more confidence (ability) talk from your client. What did you notice after you offered a posy or a bouquet summary of change talk? For one growth area, for example, perhaps you would like to find ways to strengthen the change talk you heard. (One idea is to use the questions in Table 15.1 or Handout 15.1 to review the session.)

TABLE 15.2. Definitions of Specific MI-consistent and MI-inconsistent Behaviors

Behavior	Definitions
Questions	***Closed:*** Asks for specific information, for a "yes" or "no" response, or for numeric information. ("How many hours do you watch TV?") Closed questions restrict and narrow the answers clients can provide. ***Open:*** Allows for more flexibility in responses. "What is most important to you?" or "How do you think you could do that?" "Tell me . . . " statements can also be open questions. ("Tell me how a typical day looks for you.")
Reflections	***Simple reflections:*** (SR) Essentially repeats what the client said, adding little or no meaning or emphasis beyond what was said. ***Complex reflections:*** Makes a guess and adds meaning or emphasis to what the client said (or did not say). A complex reflection conveys a deeper view of what was said, whether to emphasize a point, take the conversation in a different direction, or summarize and link to something said earlier.
MI-consistent responses	• Asking permission before giving information or advice. • Affirming and supporting; acknowledging what's positive about the person or demonstrating compassion. • Emphasizing clients' autonomy, freedom of choice, and control.
MI-inconsistent responses	• Giving advice or information without permission. • Confronting by labeling, correcting, blaming, or disagreeing. • Directing by giving orders, or otherwise challenging clients' autonomy.

MITI coding tool, by counting how often a specific skill occurs. You can listen to a recording or use a written transcript.

However, it's important to review what you are looking for so you can recognize it when you hear it. This clarity can also improve reliability and ensure that two observers produce similar observations. See Table 15.2 for summary definitions of the specific MI behaviors based on what we presented in earlier chapters. You can count responses as you listen to a live session, but for more reliable measurement, it is advisable to use the transcripts of sessions.

Suggested Competency Thresholds

How will you know you have reached the level of proficiency that is likely to result in client change if such a thing exists? The threshold for competency could vary depending on the context, and there is no predetermined

TABLE 15.3. Suggested Competency and Proficiency Thresholds

Index	Formula	Basic	Proficient
% of complex reflections	Number of complex reflections divided by total reflections	≥40%	≥50%
% of open questions	Number of open questions divided by total questions	≥50%	≥70%
Ratio of reflections to questions	Number of questions divided by number of questions	≥1.0	≥2.0

level of training that leads to skillfulness. It is best to use a set of criteria to measure your skill on two levels: basic and proficient. These are suggestions based on the experience of Miller and Rollnick (2013) and serve as a starting point. Further research may provide more specifics in gauging the skill level needed for successful change.

After you observe or listen to a recorded session, you could use the formulas in Table 15.3 to gather baseline data and, from there, develop targets for future growth.

PROFESSIONAL LEARNING COMMUNITIES

> The next best thing to being wise oneself
> is to live in a circle of those who are.
> —C. S. Lewis

Reading this book alone is unlikely to improve your skillfulness. You might gain short-term improvements by attending further training or a workshop. But to strengthen learning and grow in competence in MI, receiving objective feedback and guidance on observed practice is needed.

A professional learning community (PLC) is an excellent opportunity for ongoing professional development. Working with a group of peer coaches is based on the notion that learning is an ongoing process, and group feedback is often more beneficial than working alone (Prenger et al., 2018). In our experience, learning alongside a group of coaches is also more fun.

Growth Mindset

A growth mindset is essential for coaches. Notice how the ICF professional certified coach marker in Competency 2 echoes this: "Embodying a coaching mindset . . . that requires ongoing learning and development, establishing a reflective practice, and preparing for sessions" (IFC, 2020a). Additionally, the ICF code of ethics speaks to this in Section 2, code 16: "Commit to excellence through continued personal, professional, and ethical development" (IFC, 2022).

As a coach who helps clients reframe negativity, you are well acquainted with attitudes and perceptions that promote positive growth and learning. Here is a review.

- You view efforts as experiments, not "tests," thus alleviating the pressure to get it "right."
- You are open to opportunities for growth instead of overestimating your abilities.
- You see mistakes as opportunities to learn and grow, adopting the mindset that it's okay to be a beginner.
- You feel capable when faced with challenges instead of being self-critical.
- You welcome others' perspectives and the chance to try out your MI skills.

Learning Cycles

The learning cycle in a PLC for coaches is similar to what teachers experience working in collaborative teams (Southwest Educational Development Laboratory, 2005). An effective model includes content review, setting goals, practice, feedback, adjusting, and creating a personalized plan with new goals for growth. Here is an overview of those six steps, which recur in cycles.

1. **Content review.** Content review of MI-specific skills, spirit (the coaches' CAPE), or structure can build a platform for selecting a growth goal. This might include reviewing the content in this book or other literature and online webinars, videos, or podcasts about MI practice.
2. **Setting goals.** Setting personal and specific goals for improvement is similar to establishing a focus for coaching sessions. Selecting the desired target for your work helps the team (and you) orient the observation and feedback around your chosen goal. A good practice is to choose only one goal to focus on per session.
3. **Practice.** Practice is the deliberate, mindful way to grow beyond your current ability. It involves breaking skills into chunks and applying them at increasingly challenging levels. The objective is not to become an "expert" but to scaffold your practice so that you make increasing progress beyond your current level and have a more proficient and comfortable experience.

4. **Feedback.** Feedback confirms what you did well and how close you came to your desired goal. The most effective feedback is tied directly to your chosen goal. It's often hard to see our own practice, and having our peers help us "see" is one of the most valuable benefits of a PLC.
5. **Adjusting.** Adjusting refers to the things you would like to improve. It may mean doing less of something (giving information without permission) and more of something else (offering more complex than simple reflections). Or it could mean moving a skill from basic to proficient level.
6. **Personalized plan for new goals.** Creating a personalized plan with new goals is an excellent way to learn complex skills in MI. You might choose individual skills, such as asking evocative questions, or you might try combining skills, such as evoking to build confidence.

PRACTICAL GUIDELINES FOR PLCS

Here are some practical suggestions for setting up an effective PLC. Besides the growth mindset mentioned above, you might think of other ways to use the MI-consistent coach approach when interacting with your peer learners. For example, you continue to wear the lens of positivity to first highlight and affirm what you (or another coach from your group) did well. The list below is not the only way, but these suggestions are based on best practices for learning together.

1. Choose parameters and establish group norms that help members feel safe to take risks and keep learning.
2. Learning from peers is effective, but one caution is avoiding getting off track and developing some practice variants. Inviting a periodic check-in from a mentor or someone experienced and trained in MI is advisable. However, bring your growth and creative mindset because you may discover many ways to do MI "right."
3. Begin each session with a review of "What's gone well" since your last meeting, specifically, the MI skills you noticed in coaching that you want to acknowledge.
4. Determine the specific skill(s) that the coach wants the observers to notice and reflect on. All team members will focus their observations and feedback on that particular goal. For example, the coach may want you to focus on the number of open versus closed questions or the skill of strengthening change talk.
5. Use recorded sessions and listen in chunks of 10 minutes and then stop for feedback before starting the recording again. You might

also want to have peers coach each other, in which case it is more effective to have a "real-play" scenario instead of role play. The person playing the client talks about something they are considering or want to change.

6. You can use Boxes 15.1 and 15.2 to reflect or give feedback to your peers related to their chosen skills. All observers can look at the

BOX 15.2. Suggested Open Questions for Self-Reflection and Peer Feedback

Directions: After a coaching session, use these questions in your professional learning community as a guide for offering self-reflection and peer feedback.

SELF-REFLECTION

Suggested Open Questions for Self-Reflection

- "What do I think went well?"
- "Did it go as planned? If not, what are my thoughts about that?"
- "How do I think the client felt? Why do I say that?"
- "What did I learn from this session?"
- "If I were doing this again, what would I do the same? What would I do differently?
- "What difference might this make?"

PEER FEEDBACK

The main thing is to use open questions and give the coach the opportunity to think and reflect (not unlike coaching!). Here are some tips:

- Offer feedback as soon as possible after the event.
- Think about the coach's desired target for this session. Restrict your feedback to the chosen target.
- Create a safe environment by noticing and highlighting positives. Tell what went well.
- Be specific, and if the coach asks you directly, offer one suggestion for a way to improve.

Suggested Open Questions for Feedback

- "What do you think went well?"
- "To what extent do you feel you met your target goal?"
- "What do you think you might want to do differently?"
- "What, if anything, do you want to improve further?"
- "What are some ideas you have for how to achieve this?"

one selected goal, and if the coach chooses, they might focus on additional skills. (See also Handout 15.3 online at *www.guilford.com/lanier-materials.*)

SUGGESTED SEQUENCE FOR GIVING AND RECEIVING FEEDBACK

Box 15.3 presents a suggested sequence to follow when providing feedback in the PLC.

SELF-REFLECTION AND PEER FEEDBACK FORM

You can use the feedback form in Figure 15.1 as a template for self-reflection and providing feedback to other coaches in your PLC. (For a blank version of this form, see Handout 15.4 online at *www.guilford.com/lanier-materials.*) The form can be given to the coach and the observer(s). Figure 15.1 includes some sample responses by the coach and the observer.

BOX 15.3. Suggested Sequence for Giving and Receiving Feedback

1. The coach reflects after the session to answer questions such as "What went well?" and "What would you want more of or less of?"

2. The client (if it's a live session) reflects on what they experienced and what seemed especially helpful.

3. The observers can give feedback about what went well and use Handout 15.4, "Suggestions for Self-Reflection and Peer Feedback Form," as a guide. They might also share more objective observations if appropriate (e.g., 11 reflections to seven questions, more complex reflections than simple ones, etc.).

4. (Optional) Allow one observer to offer a recommendation or suggestion. If the coach has given permission, the suggestion could include an example of something to try next time. In alignment with the integrity of MI-consistent coaching, offering affirmations of efforts and personal strengths and capabilities goes a long way in building confidence to try new things.

5. After graciously receiving the feedback, the coach can choose one specific skill or behavior to target for the next time. For example, if there were more questions than reflections, the new goal might be to increase to at least an equal number of reflections to questions in future sessions.

Coach: *Cecilia Lanier* Observer: *Patty Bean and Stacey Arnold*

Today's Date: *12/1/23* Session Date: *11/10/23*

Coach's Target Goal: *Listening for the number of reflections per questions, and open vs. closed questions.*

BEFORE SESSION:

Identify the coach's targeted goal for this session. Ask specifically what kind of feedback the coach is requesting. The coach might ask you to look for broader components such as partnership, empathy, cultivating change talk, and softening sustain talk (refer to Table 15.1). Or the coach might want you to count specific behaviors, as in the example below (refer to Table 15.2 for definitions of specific behaviors). Record only what is requested by the coach.

DURING SESSION:

Your first goal is to focus on what the coach has chosen for observation. If the coach wants you to look at specific skills (see example below), you could count those as the session progresses. If you have a transcript of a recorded session available, you can jot notes on your copy of the transcript. Here is an example of what the peer coaches listened for and counted during the session.

- The number of questions. *13 questions asked.*
- The number of reflections. *5 reflections given.*
- The number of closed *3* versus open *10* questions.
- The number of simple *N/A* versus complex *N/A* reflections.
- The number of affirmations and other MI-consistent responses. *N/A*
- The number of MI-consistent responses. *N/A*
- The number of MI-inconsistent responses. *N/A*

(Refer to Table 15.2 for MI-consistent and MI-inconsistent responses.)

AFTER SESSION:

Coach Self-Reflection (Some suggestions for open questions to consider. Sample coach responses are provided.)

- What went well? *Most of my questions were open-ended.*
- Did it go as planned? *I'm surprised at how few reflections I gave.*
- If not, what are my thoughts? *I felt my client wasn't moving forward, so I started asking more questions.*

(continued)

FIGURE 15.1. Example of a completed Self-Reflection and Peer Feedback Form.

- How do I think the client felt? *He may have felt pressured a bit.*
- What examples might support my thoughts? *He gave short answers.*
- What did I learn from this session? *It's hard to listen to the client if I worry that they need to move on.*
- What would I do more of next time? *Use more reflections and pause more so my client would explore and talk more.*
- What would I do less of or differently next time? *Use less questions and try to stop worrying about what the client should do.*
- Why? *To help my client be more engaged and do the work. Also, I could listen better.*
- What might be a target goal to focus on next? *Increase the number of reflections to at least half of the number of questions.*

Tips for Observer Feedback

Use open questions and allow the coach time to think and reflect (much like coaching!). Here are some suggestions.

- Offer feedback as soon as possible after the event.
- Focus on the coach's desired target for this session and restrict feedback to that target unless the coach asks for more.
- Create safety and trust in the relationship by noticing and affirming what went well.
- Be specific, and if the coach asks you directly, offer ***one*** suggestion for improving.

Suggested Open Questions for Offering Feedback

- What went well? *You offered 5 pretty powerful reflections. And I noticed most of your questions were open-ended.*
- To what extent do you feel you met your target goal? *Honestly, I wasn't aware during the session of how few reflections I offered. But after today, I'll be better able to take notice of that.*
- What might you want to do differently? *I want to calm down and just listen more deeply. If I stay curious, I think I'll be better at offering reflections.*
- "What, if anything, do you want to improve further?" *I'll stay with this goal and see if I can increase the number of reflections next time.*

FIGURE 15.1. *(continued)*

A ROADMAP FOR LEARNING

Where do you start to improve MI in your coaching? The ultimate goal is to integrate the spirit (CAPE), skills, and structure of MI in a natural flow in your sessions. As suggested earlier, when you want to improve MI, it is helpful to focus on one specific component or core skill of MI at a time. Eventually, as you become more comfortable, you can try combining different skills in a more dynamic and responsive way. Here is a list of 11 of those tasks.

1. **Embrace MI spirit.** Developing and actively promoting the underlying spirit of MI (coaches' CAPE): compassion, acceptance, partnership, and empowerment (Chapter 3).
2. **Reflectively listen, OARS.** Developing and deepening reflective-listening skills and use of OARS (Chapter 4).
3. **Focus.** Partnering with clients to clarify the agenda and identify specific change goals to move toward (Chapter 5).
4. **Provide information and advice.** Sharing information and offering advice in an MI-consistent style (Chapter 8).
5. **Identify change talk and sustain talk.** Attuning your ear to recognize change talk and sustain talk (Chapter 6).
6. **Evoke.** Evoking change talk through the strategic use of OARS skills (Chapter 7).
7. **Strengthen change talk.** Responding to change talk in a way to strengthen it (Chapter 7).
8. **Soften sustain talk.** Responding to sustain talk and discord in a way to soften it, not magnify it (Chapter 9).
9. **Support hope and confidence.** Eliciting and strengthening hope and confidence and affirming positive traits (Chapter 10).
10. **Plan.** Managing the time, and also recognizing signs of readiness to plan and partnering to negotiate a change plan (Chapter 13).
11. **Strengthen commitment.** Listening for and reinforcing commitment language (Chapter 13).

Guidelines for Where to Start

What is most important for learning and improving MI? Where do you start? First, we acknowledge and encourage the integration of MI with other evidence-based methods for facilitating change and growth. You may have a prior background as a counselor or a supportive helper in another field, and you are comfortable using client-centered engaging skills. Whether or not you have this experience, you can benefit from assessing your current skill level and choosing specific learning goals. This becomes the basis for selecting the next steps for guided practice with feedback. Here are four broad components that we suggest you include in your training and professional growth plans if you want to improve your MI competency level.

1. *MI content knowledge and the MI spirit (coaches' CAPE).* This book provides foundational knowledge to build upon. Watching demonstrations of MI-consistent coaching can enhance learning either in the MI spirit or particular skills.
2. *Engaging,* especially the skill of accurate empathy, is essential for developing the container for coaching with MI. As we reviewed in Chapter 14, the OARS skills are used in the engaging task but without a goal-directed approach.
3. *Evoking* is unique to MI and, with the added component of focusing, is essential to facilitating people's change and growth. The important skills are finding a clear focus, recognizing, evoking, and responding to change talk in ways to strengthen it.
4. *Planning* includes the negotiation of a change plan. The skills to focus on are timing (knowing when the client is ready), creating a plan, and evoking commitment. These skills are integrated with other evidence-based practices that facilitate and encourage the successful implementation of change goals.

SUMMARY

Skillfulness in MI is developed over time with ongoing feedback and coaching based on observed practice. Becoming proficient in MI-consistent coaching is worth celebrating. But the real test of success is whether clients actually change. Broadly, we know that over 2,500 randomized clinical trials have studied the effectiveness of MI in various fields and that specific tools have been developed to measure the quality of MI delivered. Positive effects of MI are reported across a wide range of change goals.

MI is continually developing, and new studies and advances will likely continue to validate and improve its effectiveness in coaching. Though MI has spread into various fields of service, we believe it aligns seamlessly with coaching and becomes not only an adjacent method but a foundational bedrock for the entire coaching paradigm.

References

Acha, K. (2023, April 10). Three types of goals. *www.kennethacha.com/three-types-of-goals.*

Ambrose, S., Bridges, M., Lovett, M., DiPietro, M., & Norman, M. (2010). *How learning works: Seven research-based principles for smart teaching.* Jossey-Bass.

Amrhein, P. C., Miller, W. R., Yahne, C. E., Palmer, M., & Fulcher, L. (2003). Client commitment language during motivational interviewing predicts drug use outcomes. *Journal of Consulting and Clinical Psychology, A71*(5), 862–878.

Apodaca, T. R., Borsari, B., Jackson, K. M., Magill, M., Longabaugh, R., Mastroleo, N. R., & Barnett, N. P. (2014). Sustain talk predicts poorer outcomes among mandated college student drinkers receiving a brief motivational intervention. *Psychology of Addictive Behaviors, 28*(3), 631–638.

Apodaca, T. R., Jackson, K. M., Borsari, B., Magill, M., Longabaugh, R., Mastroleo, N. R., & Barnett, N. P. (2016). Which individual therapist behaviors elicit client change talk and sustain talk in motivational interviewing? *Journal of Substance Abuse Treatment, 61*, 60–65.

Arloski, M. (2014). *Wellness coaching for lasting lifestyle change.* Whole Person Associates.

Bandura, A. (1997). *Self-efficacy: The exercise of control.* Freeman.

Bandura, A. (2000). Exercise of human agency through collective efficacy. *Current Directions in Psychological Science, 9*(3), 75–78.

Bandura, A. (2008). Toward an agentic theory of the self. *Advances in Self Research, 3*, 15–49.

Bandura, A., & Cervone, D. (1983). Self-evaluative and self-efficacy mechanisms governing the motivational effects of goal systems. *Journal of Personality and Social Psychology, 45*, 1017–1028.

Baron, L., & Morin, L. (2012). The working alliance in executive coaching: Its impact on outcomes and how coaches can influence it. In E. de Haan & C. Sills (Eds.), *Coaching relationships* (pp. 213–226). Libri.

Benzo, R. P. (2013). Mindfulness and motivational interviewing: two candidate methods for promoting self-management. *Chronic Respiratory Disease, 10*(3), 175–182.

Boehmer, K. R., Álvarez-Villalobos, N. A., Barakat, S., de Leon-Gutierrez, H., Ruiz-Hernandez, F. G., Elizondo-Omaña, G. G., . . . Wang, Z. (2023). The impact of health and wellness coaching on patient-important outcomes in chronic illness care: A systematic review and meta-analysis. *Patient Education and Counseling, 117*, Article 107975.

Bohart, A. C., & Tallman, K. (2010). Clients: The neglected common factor in psychotherapy. In B. L. Duncan, S. D. Miller, B. E. Wampold, & M. A. Hubble (Eds.), *The heart and soul of change: Delivering what works in therapy* (2nd ed., pp. 83–111). American Psychological Association.

Boyatzis, R., Smith, M. L., & Oosten, V. E. (2019). *Helping people change: Coaching with compassion for lifelong learning and growth.* Harvard Business Review Press.

Brehm, S. S., & Brehm, J. W. (2013). *Psychological reactance: A theory of freedom and control.* Academic Press.

Brinks, J., Fowler, A., Franklin, B. A., & Dulai, J. (2017). Lifestyle modification in secondary prevention: Beyond pharmacotherapy. *American Journal of Lifestyle Medicine, A11*(2), 137–152.

Brown, J. M. (1998). Self-regulation and the addictive behaviors. In W. R. Miller & N. Heather (Eds.), *Treating addictive behaviors* (2nd ed., pp. 61–74). Plenum Press.

Centers for Disease Control and Prevention. (2020b). National diabetes statistics report, 2020. Available at *www.cdc.gov/diabetes/library/features/diabetes-stat-report.html.*

Chariyeva, Z., Golin, C. E., Earp, J. A., Maman, S., Suchindran, C., & Zimmer, C. (2013). The role of self-efficacy and motivation to explain the effect of motivational interviewing time on changes in risky sexual behavior among people living with HIV: A mediation analysis. *AIDS and Behavior,17*, 813–823.

Cialdini, R. (2007). *Influence: The psychology of persuasion.* HarperCollins.

Clark, M. M., Bradley, K. L., Jenkins, S. M., Mettler, E. A., Larson, B. G., Preston, H. R., . . . Harris, A. M. (2014). The effectiveness of wellness coaching for improving quality of life. *Mayo Clinic Proceedings, 89*(11), 1537–1544.

Clifford, D., & Curtis, L. (2016). *Motivational interviewing in nutrition and fitness.* Guilford Press.

Critcher, C. R., Duning, D., & Armor, D. A. (2010. When self-affirmations reduce defensiveness: Timing is key. *Personality and Social Psychology Bulletin, 36*(7), 947–959.

Crits-Christoph, P., Hamilton, J. L., Ring-Kurtz, S. R. G., McClure, B., Kulaga, A., & Rotrosen, J. (2011). Program, counselor, and patient variability in the alliance: A multilevel study of the alliance in relation to substance use outcomes. *Journal of Substance Abuse Treatment, 40*(4), 405–413.

Cummins, R. A. (2013). *Subjective well-being homeostasis.* Oxford Bibliographies Online Datasets.

de Almeida Neto, A. C. (2017). Understanding motivational interviewing: An evolutionary perspective. *Evolutionary Psychological Science, 3*(4), 379–389.

De Haan, E. (2011). *Relational coaching: Journeys towards mastering one-to-one learning.* Wiley.

De Haan, E., Culpin, V., & Curd, J. (2011). Executive coaching in practice: What determines helpfulness for clients of coaching? *Personnel Review, 40*(1), 24–44.

Deci, E. D., & Ryan, R. (1985). *Intrinsic motivation and self-determination in human behavior.* Plenum Press.

Deci, E. L., & Ryan, R. M. (2013). The importance of autonomy for development and well-being. In B. Sokol, F. M. E. Grouzet, & U. Muller (Eds.), *Self-regulation and autonomy: Social, developmental, educational, and neurological dimensions of human contact* (pp. 19–46). Cambridge University Press.

DiClemente, C. C., Bellino, L. E., & Neavins, T. M. (1999). Motivation for change and alcoholism treatment. *Alcohol Research & Health, 23*(2), 86–92.

Dueease, B. (2009). The history of life coaching. Available at *https://findyourcoach.com/wilc/the-history-of-life-coaching.*

Elliott, R., Bohart, A. C., Watson, J. C., & Greenberg, L. S. (2011). Empathy. In J. C. Norcross (Ed.), *Psychotherapy relationships that work: Evidence-based responsiveness* (2nd ed., pp. 132–152). Oxford University Press.

Elliott, R., Bohart, A. C., Watson, J. C., & Murphy, D. (2018). Therapist empathy and client outcome: An updated meta-analysis. *Psychotherapy, 55*, 399–410.

ESV study bible. (2016). Crossway.

Flückiger, C., Rubel, J., Del Re, A. C., Horvath, A. O., Wampold, B. E., Crits-Christoph, P., . . . Barber, J. P. (2020). The reciprocal relationship between alliance and early treatment symptoms: A two-stage individual participant data meta-analysis. *Journal of Consulting and Clinical Psychology, 88*(9), 829–843.

Frates, E. P., Moore, M. A., Lopez, C. N, & McMahon, G. T. (2011). Coaching for behavior change in physiatry. *American Journal of Physical Medicine and Rehabilitation, 90*(12), 1074–1082.

Gaume, J., Bertholet, N., Faouzi, M., Gmel, G., & Daeppen, J. B. (2010, Oct). Counselor motivational interviewing skills and young adult change talk articulation during brief motivational interventions. *Journal of Substance Abuse Treatment, 39*(3), 272–281.

Glynn, L. H., & Moyers, T. B. (2010). Chasing change talk: The clinician's role in evoking client language about change. *Journal of Substance Abuse Treatment, 39*(1), 65–70.

Goble, K. L., Knight, S. M., Burke, S. C., Carawan, L. W., & Wolever, R. Q. (2017). Transformative change to "a new me": A qualitative study of clients' lived experience with integrative health coaching. *Coaching: An International Journal of Theory, Research and Practice, 10*(1), 18–36.

Goldhaber, D., Lavery, L., & Theobald, R. (2015). Uneven playing field? Assessing the teacher quality gap between advantaged and disadvantaged students. *Educational Researcher, 44*(5), 293–307.

Gollwitzer, P. M. (1999). Implementation intentions: Strong effects of simple plans. *American Psychologist, 54*(7), 493–503.

Gordon, T. (1970). *P.E.T., parent effectiveness training: The tested new way to raise responsible children.* Wyden.

Hardavella, G., Aamli-Gaagnat, A., Saad, N., Rousalova, I., & Sreter, K. B. (2017). How to give and receive feedback effectively. *Breathe, 13*(4), 327–333.

Harvard Graduate School of Education. (2012, November 2). Atul Gawande: The difference between coaching and teaching [Video]. YouTube. Available at *www.youtube.com/watch?v=VabtGPVVihA.*

Hashemzadeh, M., Rahimi, A., Zare-Farashbandi, F., Alavi-Naeini, A. M., & Daei, A. (2019). Transtheoretical model of health behavioral change: A systematic review. *Iranian Journal of Nursing and Midwifery Research, 24*(2), 83–90.

Hatfield, E., Cacioppo, J. T., & Rapson, R. L. (1993). Emotional contagion. *Current Directions in Psychological Science, 2*(3), 96–100.

Hill, C. (2009). *Helping skills: Facilitating exploration, insight and action* (3rd ed.). American Psychological Association.

Hojat, M., DeSantis, J., Shannon, S. C., Mortensen, L. H., Speicher, M. R., Bragan, L., . . . Calabrese, L. H. (2018). The Jefferson Scale of Empathy: A nationwide study of measurement properties, underlying components, latent variable structure, and national norms in medical students. *Advances in Health Sciences Education: Theory and Practice, 23*(5), 899–920.

Horvath, A., Fluckiger, C., Del Re, A., & Symonds, D. (2011). Alliance in individual psychotherapy. *Psychotherapy (Chic), 48*(1), 9–16.

Howard, A. R. (2015). Coaching to vision versus coaching to improvement needs: A preliminary investigation on the differential impacts of fostering positive and negative emotion during real time executive coaching sessions. *Frontiers in Psychology, 6*, 455.

Hubble, M., Duncan, B., & Miller, S. (Eds.). (1999). *The heart and soul of change: What works in therapy.* American Psychological Association.

International Coaching Federation. (2007). What is coaching? Available at *www.coachfederation.org.*

International Coaching Federation. (2019). ICF core competencies. Available at *https://coachingfederation.org/credentials-and-standards/core-competencies.*

International Coaching Federation. (2020a). PCC (professional certified coach) markers. Available at *https://coachingfederation.org/credentials-and-standards/performance-evaluations/pcc-markers.*

International Coaching Federation. (2020b). 2020 ICF global coaching study: Executive summary 3. Available at *https://coachfederation.org/app/uploads/2020/09/FINAL_ICF_GCS2020_ExecutiveSummary.pdf.*

International Coaching Federation. (2022). ICF code of ethics. Available at *https://coachingfederation.org/ethics/code-of-ethics.*

Ivey, A. E., Ivey, M. B., & Zalaquett, C. P. (2009). *Intentional interviewing and counseling* (7th ed.). Brooks/Cole.

Jordan, M. (2022). *How to be a health coach* (3rd ed.). Global Medicine Enterprises.

Karno, M., & Longabaugh, R. (2005). An examination of how therapist directiveness interacts with patient anger and reactance to predict alcohol use. *Journal of Studies on Alcohol, 66*(6), 825–832.

Kimsey-House, K., Kimsey-House, H., Sandhal, P., & Whitworth, L. (2018). *Co-active coaching: The proven framework for transformative conversations at work and in life* (4th ed.). Nicholas Brealey.

Lancha, A. H., Jr., Sforzo, G. A., & Pereira-Lancha, L. O. (2018). Improving nutritional habits with no diet prescription: Details of a nutritional coaching process. *American Journal of Lifestyle Medicine, 12*(2), 160–165.

LeDoux, J. E. (2020, June 8). Thoughtful feelings. *Current Biology, 30*, Article 617–635. Available at *www.cell.com/current-biology/pdf/S0960-9822(20)30492-9.pdf.*

Luborsky, L., Crits-Christoph, P., Alexander, L., Margolis, M., & Cohen, M. (1983). Two helping alliance methods for predicting outcomes of psychotherapy. *Journal of Nervous and Mental Disease, A171*(8), 480–491.

Magill, M., Apodaca, T. R., Borsari, B., Gaume, J., Hoadley, A., Gordon, R. E. F., . . . Moyers, T. (2018). A meta-analysis of motivational interviewing process: Technical, relational, and conditional process models of change. *Journal of Consulting and Clinical Psychology, 86*(2), 140–157.

Magill, M., Bernstein, M. H., Hoadley, A., Borsari, B., Apodaca, T. R., Gaume, J., & Tonigan, J. S. (2019). Do what you say and say what you are going to do: A preliminary meta-analysis of client change and sustain talk subtypes in motivational interviewing. *Psychotherapy Research, 29*(7), 860–869.

Magill, M., Stout, R. L., & Apodaca, T. R. (2013). Therapist focus on ambivalence and commitment: A longitudinal analysis of motivational interviewing treatment ingredients. *Psychology of Addictive Behaviors, 27*(3), 754–762.

Marcdante, K., & Simpson, D. (2018). Choosing when to advise, coach, or mentor. *Journal of Graduate Medical Education, A10*(2), 227–228.

McClintock, A. S., Anderson, T. M., Anderson, C. L., & Wing, E. H. (2019). Early psychotherapeutic empathy, alliance, and client outcome: Preliminary evidence of indirect effects. *Journal of Clinical Psychology, 74*, 839–848.

McGregor, D., & Cutcher-Gershenfeld, J. (2006). *The human side of enterprise, annotated edition.* McGraw Hill Professional.

Miller, W. R. (1983). Motivational interviewing with problem drinkers. *Behavioral Psychotherapy, 11*, 147–172.

Miller, W. R. (2022). *On second thought: How ambivalence shapes your life.* Guilford Press.

Miller, W. R., & Moyers, T. B. (2021). *Effective psychotherapists: Clinical skills that improve client outcomes.* Guilford Press.

Miller, W. R., & Rollnick, S. (1992). *Motivational interviewing: Preparing people to change addictive behavior.* Guilford Press.

Miller, W. R., & Rollnick, S. (2002). *Motivational interviewing: Preparing people for change* (2nd ed.). Guilford Press.

Miller, W. R., & Rollnick, S. (2013). *Motivational interviewing: Helping people change* (3rd ed.). Guilford Press.

Miller, W. R., & Rollnick, S. (2023). *Motivational interviewing: Helping people change and grow* (4th ed.). Guilford Press.

Miller, W. R., Rollnick, S., & Moyers, T. B. (2019). *Motivational interviewing: AFoundational online course.* Psychwire.

Miller, W. R., & Rose, G. S. (2015). Motivational interviewing and decisional balance: Contrasting responses to client ambivalence. *Behavioural and Cognitive Psychotherapy, 43*(2), 129–141.

Miller, W. R., Taylor, C. A., & West, J. C. (1980). Focused versus broad-spectrum behavior therapy for problem drinkers. *Journal of Consulting and Clinical Psychology, 48*, 590–601.

Mohr, D. C. (1995). Negative outcome in psychotherapy: A critical review. *Clinical Science and Practice, 2*(1), 1–27.

Moore, C. (2019). Learned optimism: Is Martin Seligman's glass half full? *Positive Psychology.* Available at *https://positivepsychology.com/learned-optimism.*

Moore, M., Jackson, E., & Tschannen-Noran, B., (2016) *Coaching psychology manual.* Wolters Kluwer.

Moyers, T. B., & Martin, T. (2006). Therapist influence on client language during motivational interviewing sessions. *Journal of Substance Abuse Treatment, 30*(3), 245–251.

Moyers, T. B., Martin, T., Houck, J. M., Christopher, P. J., & Tonigan, J. S. (2009). From in-session behaviors to drinking outcomes: A causal chain for motivational interviewing. *Journal of Consulting and Clinical Psychology, 77*(6), 1113–1124.

Moyers, T. B., & Miller, W. R. (2013). Is low therapist empathy toxic? *Psychology of Addictive Behaviors, 27*(3), 878–884.

National Board for Health and Wellness Coaching. (2017). NBHWC code of ethics. Available at *https://nbhwc.org/code-of-ethics.*

National Board for Health and Wellness Coaching. (2020, June). NBHWC program approval published standards. Available at *https://nbhwc.org/program-approval-standards.*

National Board for Health and Wellness Coaching. (2021). Scope of practice. Available at *https://nbhwc.org/scope-of-practice.*

National Board for Health and Wellness Coaching. (2022). NBHWC practical skills guidelines. Available at *https://nbhwc.org/program-approval-standards.*

National Board of Medical Examiners & National Board for Health and Wellness Coaching. (2022). Health and wellness coach certifying examination. Available at *www.nbme.org/sites/default/files/2022-05/HWCCE_Bulletin_of_Information.pdf.*

Norcross, J. C., & Wampold, B. E. (2011). Evidence-based therapy relationships: Research conclusions and clinical practices. *Psychotherapy, 48*(1), 98–102.

Norcross, J. C., & Wampold, B. E. (2018). A new therapy for each patient: Evidence-based relationships and responsiveness. *Journal of Clinical Psychology, 74*(11), 1889–1906.

O'Hara, D. (2017). The intrinsic motivation of Richard Ryan and Edward Deci. Available at *www.apa.org/members/content/intrinsic-motivation.*

Oxford Languages. (2022). Oxford languages and Google. Available at *https://languages.oup.com/google-dictionary-en.*

Page, N., & de Haan, E. (2014). Does executive coaching work? *The Psychologist,* 27(8).

Parry, C., Kramer, H. M., & Coleman, E. A. (2006). A qualitative exploration of a patient-centered coaching intervention to improve care transitions in chronically ill older adults. *Home Health Care Services Quarterly, 25*(3–4), 39–53.

Prenger, R., Poortman, C. L., & Handelzalts, A. (2018). The effects of networked professional learning communities. *Journal of Teacher Education, A70*(5), 441–452.

Prochaska, J. O. (1994). Strong and weak principles for progressing from precontemplation to action on the basis of twelve problem behaviors. *Health Psychology, 13,* 47–51.

Prochaska, J. O., DiClemente, C. C., & Norcross, J. C. (1992). In search of how people change: Applications to addictive behaviors. *American Psychologist, 47*(9), 1102–1114.

Prochaska, J. O., Norcross, J. C., & DiClemente, C. C. (1994). *Changing for good: The revolutionary program that explains the six stages of change and teaches you how to free yourself from bad habits.* Avon Books.

Prochaska, J. O., & Prochaska, J. M. (2016). *Changing to thrive: Using the stages of change to overcome the top threats to your health and happiness.* Simon and Schuster.

Ragone, I., & Seaborne, S. (2016, December 16). Shay Seaborne, CPTSD, trauma awareness activist-artist [Video]. Available at *www.shayseaborne.com.*

Rankins, N. C. (2016, May 15). Your patient should get a health coach. Here's why. *KevinMD.com.* Available at *www.kevinmd.com/2016/05/your-patient-should-get-a-health-coach-heres-why.html.*

Reid, A. E., Cialdini, R. B., & Aiken, L. S. (2010). Social norms and health behavior. In A. Steptoe (Ed.), *Handbook of behavioral medicine: Methods and approaches* (pp. 263–274). Springer.

Rogers, C. R. (1951). *Client-centered therapy.* Houghton Mifflin.

Rogers, C. R. (1980). *A way of being.* Houghton Mifflin.

Ryan, R. M., & Deci, E. L. (2000). Self-determination theory and the facilitation of intrinsic motivation, social development, and well-being. *The American Psychologist, 55*(1), 68–78.

Ryan, R. M., & Deci, E. L. (2008). A self-determination theory approach to psychotherapy: The motivational basis for effective change. *Canadian Psychology/Psychologie Canadienne, 49*(3), 186–193.

Safran, J. D., McMain, S., Murray, P., & Crocker, P. (1990). Therapeutic alliance rupture as a therapy event for empirical investigation. *Psychotherapy: Theory, Research, Practice, Training, 27*(2), 154–165.

Schunk, D. H. (1995). Self-efficacy, motivation, and performance. *Journal of Applied Sport Psychology, 7*(2), 112–137.

Seligman, M. E. P. (2006). *Learned optimism: How to change your mind and your life.* Vintage.

Seltzer, L. F. (2019). The rebellion of the over-criticized: A child's rebellion against too-strict parents can lead to self-sabotage. Available at *www.psychologytoday.com/us/blog/evolution-the-self/201904/the-rebellion-the-over-criticized-child.*

Shahnazari, M., Ceresa, C., Foley, S., Fong, A., Zidaru, E., & Moody, S. (2013). Nutrition-focused wellness coaching promotes a reduction in body weight in overweight U.S. veterans. *Journal of the Academy of Nutrition and Dietetics, 113*(7), 928–935.

Shearn, D. (2001). Commentary: Changing physician behavior: What does it take? *Western Journal of Medicine, 175*(3), 167.

Sherman, S., & Freas, A. (2004). The Wild West of executive coaching. *Harvard Business Review, A82*(11), 82–90.

Sime, C., & Jacob, Y. (2018). Crossing the line? A qualitative exploration of ICF master certified: Coaches' perception of roles, borders and boundaries. *International Coaching Psychology Review, 13*(2), 46–61.

Smither, J. W., London, M., Flautt, R., Vargas, Y., & Kucine, I. (2003). Can working with an executive coach improve multisource feedback ratings over time? A quasi-experimental field study. *Personnel Psychology, 56*, 23–44.

Southwest Educational Development Laboratory. (2005). The professional teaching and learning cycle: Introduction. Available at *https://sedl.org/txcc/resources/working_systemically/ptlc-intro.pdf*.

Spence, G. B., & Oades, L. G. (2011). Coaching with determination in mind: Using theory to advance evidence-based coaching practice. *International Journal of Evidence Based Coaching and Mentoring, 9*(2).

Steyn, Dr. D. (Host). (2022, April 8). Q&A with health coach Cecilia Lanier: Health benefits of having a coach. (203) [Audio podcast episode]. Wellness MD, The Podcast. Available at *www.buzzsprout.com/1789064/10233880-q-a-with-health-coach-cecilia-lanier- health-benefits-of-having-a-coach?t=0*.

Theeboom, T., Beersma, B., & van Vianen, A. E. (2014). Does coaching work? A meta-analysis on the effects of coaching on individual level outcomes in an organizational context. *Journal of Positive Psychology, 9*(1), 1–18.

Thigpen, M. L., Beauclair, T. J., Keiser, G. M., & Guevara, M. (2007). A guide for probation and parole, motivating offenders to change. US Department of Justice, National Institute of Corrections. Available at *https://s3.amazonaws.com/static.nicic.gov/Library/022253.pdf*.

Tryon, G. S., & Winograd, G. (2011). Goal consensus and collaboration. *Psychotherapy (Chicago, Ill.), 48*(1), 50–57.

Vale, M. J., Jelinek M. V., Best J. D., Dart A. M., Grigg L. E., Hare D. L., . . . McNeil J. J. (2003). Coaching patients on achieving cardiovascular health (COACH). *Archives of Internal Medicine, 163*, 2775–2783.

Valle, S. K. (1981). Interpersonal functioning of alcoholism counselors and treatment outcome. *Journal of Studies on Alcohol, 42*, 783–790.

VIA Institute. (n.d.). VIA character strengths survey and character reports. Available at *www.viacharacter.org*.

Waldron, H. B., Miller, W. R., & Tonigan, J. S. (2001). Client anger as a predictor of differential response to treatment. In R. Longabaugh & P. W. Wirtz (Eds.), *Project MATCH hypotheses: Results and causal chain analyses* (pp. 134–148). National Institute on Alcohol Abuse and Alcoholism.

Wan, T., Kattan, W., & Terry, A. (2018). Health coaching and motivational interventions for diabetes and hypertension care. *International Archives of Nursing Health Care, 4*(4), 113.

Webster, L. A. (2020, December 22). Health and wellness coaches are fairly new. Here's what you need to know about them. *Washingtonpost.com*. Retrieved March 22, 2024, from *www.washingtonpost.com/lifestyle/wellness/health-wellness-coach-new/2020/12/21/0f0b239e-40ab-11eb-8db8-395dedaaa036_story.html*.

Webster, L. A. (2021, March 15). What a health coach can do for you. *BottomLineInc*. Available at *https://bottomlineinc.com/health/wellness/what-a-health-coach-can-do-for-you*.

Webster, L. A. (2022). Health and wellness coaching: "How can we support more comprehensive approaches to health care?" *NBME*. Available at *www.reassessthefuture.org/health-and-wellness-coaching-how-can-we-support-more-comprehensive-approaches-to-health-care*.

Weiner, B. (2018). The legacy of an attribution approach to motivation and emotion: A no-crisis zone. *Motivation Science, 4*(1), 4–14.

Wellness Associates, Inc. (2018). *Key concept #1: The illness–wellness continuum.* The Wellspring. Available at *www.thewellspring.com/wellspring/introduction-to-wellness/357/key-concept-1-the-illnesswellness-continuum.cfm.html.*

White, W. L., & Miller, W. R. (2007). The use of confrontation in addiction treatment: History, science, and time for a change. *The Counselor, A8*(4), 12–30.

Williams, P., & Menendez, D. S. (2023). *Becoming a professional life coach: The art and science of a whole-person approach* (3rd ed.). Norton.

Wolever, R. Q., Dreusicke, M., Fikkan, J., Hawkins, T. V., Yeung, S., Wakefield, J., . . . Skinner, J. (2010). Integrative health coaching for patients with type 2 diabetes. *The Diabetes Educator, 36*(4), 629–639.

Wolever, R. Q., Simmons, L. A., Sforzo, G. A., Dill, D., Kaye, M., Bechard, E. M., . . . Yang, N. (2013). A systematic review of the literature on health and wellness coaching: defining a key behavioral intervention in healthcare. *Global Advances in Health and Medicine,* 2(4), 38–57.

Worthen, V., & Isakson, R. (2010). Hope—The anchor of the soul: Cultivating hope and positive expectancy. *Issues in Religion and Psychotherapy, 33*(1), Article 9. Available at *https://scholarsarchive.byu.edu/irp/vol33/iss1/9.*

Yang, J., Bauer, B. A., Lindeen, S. A., Perlman, A. I., Abu Dabrh, A. M., Boehmer, K. R., . . . Cutshall, S. M. (2020). Current trends in health coaching for chronic conditions: A systematic review and meta-analysis of randomized controlled trials. *Medicine, 99*(30), e21080.

Young, D. I. (2021, March 11). How to tell if your coach is worth the investment. Forbes Coaches Council, Council Post. Available at *www.forbes.com/sites/forbescoachescouncil/2021/03/11/how-to-tell-if-your-coach-is-worth-the-investment.*

Index

Note. *t* or *f* after a page number indicates a table or a figure.